SURGICAL EMERGENCIES

CONTEMPORARY ISSUES IN SMALL ANIMAL PRACTICE VOLUME 2

Editorial Advisory Board

SURGICAL EMERGENCIES

Edited by

Ronald M. Bright, D.V.M., M.S.

Diplomate American College of Veterinary Surgeons
Professor and Director of Surgical Services
Department of Urban Practice
College of Veterinary Medicine
University of Tennessee
Knoxville, Tennessee

Churchill Livingstone
New York, Edinburgh, London, Melbourne   1986

Acquisitions editor: *Gene C. Kearn*
Copy editor: *Kamely Dahir*
Production designer: *Rosalie Marcus*
Production supervisor: *Jane Grochowski*
Compositor: *Maryland Composition Company, Inc.*
Printer/Binder: *The Maple-Vail Book Manufacturing Group*

Accurate indications, adverse reactions, and dosage schedules for drugs are provided in this book, but it is possible that they may change. The reader is urged to review the package information data of the manufacturers of the medications mentioned.

Distributed in the United Kingdom by Churchill Livingstone, Robert Stevenson House, 1-3 Baxter's Place, Leith Walk, Edinburgh EH1 3AF and by associated companies, branches and representatives throughout the world.

First published 1986

Printed in U.S.A.

ISBN 0-443-08362-2

9 8 7 6 5 4 3 2 1

Library of Congress Cataloging in Publication Data
Main entry under title:

Surgical emergencies.

  (Contemporary issues in small animal practice ; v. 2)
  Includes bibliographies and index.
  1. Veterinary surgical emergencies. I. Bright,
Ronald M. II. Series. [DNLM: 1. Emergencies—
veterinary. 2. Surgery, Operative—veterinary.
W1 C0769MRW v.2 / SF 911 S961]
SF914.3.S87 1986   636.089'7026   85-22365
ISBN 0-443-08362-2

Manufactured in the United States of America

This book is dedicated to
my wife, Jan, and our children, Ryan and Lisa

Contributors

Norman Ackerman, D.V.M. Diplomate American College of Veterinary Radiologists; Associate Professor of Veterinary Radiology, College of Veterinary Medicine, University of Florida, Gainesville, Florida

Stephen J. Birchard, D.V.M., M.S. Diplomate American College of Veterinary Surgeons; Assistant Professor of Small Animal Surgery, Department of Veterinary Clinical Sciences, College of Veterinary Medicine, Ohio State University, Columbus, Ohio

Ronald M. Bright, D.V.M., M.S. Diplomate American College of Veterinary Surgeons; Professor and Director of Surgical Services, Department of Urban Practice, College of Veterinary Medicine, University of Tennessee, Knoxville, Tennessee

Erick L. Egger, D.V.M. Diplomate American College of Veterinary Surgeons; Associate Professor of Surgery, Department of Clinical Sciences, College of Veterinary Medicine and Biomedical Sciences, Colorado State University, Fort Collins, Colorado

Gary W. Ellison, D.V.M., M.S. Diplomate American College of Veterinary Surgeons; Assistant Professor of Surgical Sciences, College of Veterinary Medicine, University of Florida, Gainesville, Florida

Roger B. Fingland, D.V.M. Resident in Small Animal Surgery, Department of Veterinary Clinical Sciences, College of Veterinary Medicine, Ohio State University, Columbus, Ohio

John A. E. Hubbell, D.V.M., M.S. Diplomate American College of Veterinary Anesthesiologists; Assistant Professor and Chief of Veterinary Anesthesiology, Department of Veterinary Clinical Sciences, College of Veterinary Medicine, Ohio State University, Columbus, Ohio

Curtis W. Probst, D.V.M. Diplomate American College of Veterinary Surgeons; Assistant Professor of Small Animal Surgery, Department of Small Animal

Clinical Sciences, Veterinary Clinical Center, Michigan State University, East Lansing, Michigan

Marc R. Raffe, D.V.M., M.S. Diplomate American College of Veterinary Anesthesiologists; Associate Professor of Comparative Anesthesiology, College of Veterinary Medicine, University of Minnesota, St. Paul, Minnesota

Daniel C. Richardson, D.V.M. Diplomate American College of Veterinary Surgeons; Assistant Professor of Surgery, Department of Companion Animals and Special Species Medicine, School of Veterinary Medicine, North Carolina State University, Raleigh, North Carolina

Crispin P. Spencer, D.V.M. Diplomate American College of Veterinary Radiologists; Associate Professor of Veterinary Radiology, College of Veterinary Medicine, University of Florida, Gainesville, Florida

Preface

The objective of this timely volume in the Contemporary Issues in Small Animal Practice series is to bring together widespread information that will help the veterinarian cope better with surgical emergencies. This volume goes beyond the "state of the art surgical technique" philosophy to incorporate some important pre-, post-, and perioperative metabolic changes that force us to extend our treatment beyond the operating room. When the emergency surgical patient finally gets to the operating room, it is imperative that we recognize further derangements these patients will undergo because of the anesthetic episode and surgical experience. Recognizing this, we can then better prepare for any eventual problem that may arise.

In *Surgical Emergencies* an overview of surgical diseases related to several systems is presented ranging from diagnosis to definitive medical and surgical therapy. It is safe to predict that this book will be useful to practitioners, residents, and specialists. For the medically oriented veterinarian, it will be a refresher text in the area of emergency medicine; for the surgeon, it will afford comprehensive information useful in the management of both medical and surgical problems of the emergency patient.

I gratefully acknowledge the contributions of each of my colleagues who have written up-to-date and comprehensive chapters related to the emergency surgical patient. The concerted effort of this group of experts has resulted in a book that hopefully will enhance optimal care of our patients in need of emergency surgery.

Ronald M. Bright, D.V.M., M.S.

Contents

1 | Metabolic Response of the Emergency Surgical Patient

Ronald M. Bright

A stressful stimulus applied to an animal results in a variety of metabolic and endocrine responses. These responses vary in severity, depending on the insult. For example, a minimal response follows a simple skin incision, whereas a more complex response follows shock or major surgery. When the patient's homeostatic mechanisms are overwhelmed by too many stimuli, an insufficient response may result, allowing disequilibrium to predominate. The events we are most concerned about in our surgical patients include such things as hypovolemia, hypothermia, general anesthesia, major surgery, nonsurgical trauma, psychic stresses, and sepsis.

The response that the animal makes to a stressful stimulus has basic factors that are common to the wide spectrum of insult. In most patients, the response is maintained adequately until the pretrauma status is regained. Pathways connecting the hypothalamus to other regions of the brain enhance the integrative capacity of the hypothalamus in the sympathetic response to a wide variety of surgically related stimuli such as pain, blood pressure changes, hypercarbia, hypoxia, fear, and hypo- or hyperthermia. Sympathetic nerve fibers are present in most tissues, including endocrine glands.[5]

The adrenal medulla is a large collection of cells similar to sympathetic ganglionic neurons.[5] Stimulation of this large ganglion triggers an outpouring of epinephrine or norepinephrine. The major portion of norepinephrine is primarily released from sympathetic nerve endings that respond to increased sympathetic discharge.

Moderate surgical trauma causes a transient rise of catecholamines in the blood which is sustained for 24–48 hours.[11] Norepinephrine is usually produced in excess and takes this long to undergo degradation or re-uptake by the nerve endings.[5]

It is favorable for the animal that the catecholamine response is short-lived.[23] Should catecholamine levels remain elevated for a prolonged period of time, deleterious effects such as exhaustion of energy stores and ischemia of cellular tissues may occur.

The response of the sympathetic nervous system is diffuse.[5] Specificity as to its effect is accomplished by the existence of two types of adrenergic receptors designated *alpha* and *beta*. Norepinephrine and epinephrine have both alpha and beta properties with one type being predominant, depending on the tissue. The major effect of alpha receptors in response to trauma is vasoconstriction. This vasoconstriction to the skin, adipose tissue, kidneys, and splanchnic bed preserves blood flow to more vital structures, including the heart and brain. Beta receptor effects of importance include β_1 responses such as increased heart rate, myocardial contractility, and conduction velocity. Noncardiogenic β_2 responses include bronchial relaxation, glycogenolysis and lipolysis.[5] Epinephrine's major function is to cause vasoconstriction and to increase heart rate and cardiac contractility. Norepinephrine has its principal effect on the vasomotor activity of the smooth muscles of blood vessels, which results in vasoconstriction throughout the body, except for the myocardium.[23]

The initial response of the neuroendocrine system to stress results from hormonal changes that attempt to maintain the survival of the animal. Catecholamines are considered the primal endocrine response to injury.[23] Almost immediately upon injury, sympathetic discharge mediates hormonal and metabolic changes in at least three ways: (1) The central initiation of the hypothalamus–pituitary peripheral gland cascade depends largely on catecholamines. For example, catecholamines stimulate the pituitary, producing adrenocorticotrophic hormone (ACTH), and subsequently increase glucocorticoid and aldosterone levels. Gluconeogenesis and a shift of potassium from intracellular to extracellular spaces results.[10] (2) The pancreatic islets are modulated partly by sympathetic nerve activity in response to trauma, which influences insulin and glucagon secretion. (3) The direct metabolic effect on certain tissues is known to exist. For example, epinephrine promotes lipolysis of adipose tissue, resulting in an increase in nonesterified fatty acids (NEFA). Gluconeogenesis caused by catecholamines causes increased blood glucose levels as well. The effect of epinephrine on muscle, to inhibit the rate of glucose uptake, is partly responsible for the increased glucose levels.[5] Although at present the mechanism is unclear, norepinephrine probably mediates the sharp rise in ACTH and cortisol that is observed following injury.

The sympathetic system plays an important role in response to trauma. However, some studies have suggested benefit from inhibiting beta adrenergic responses.[33] In experimental shock produced by hemorrhage or endotoxin injection, a beta blocker, propranolol, has resulted in fewer deaths.[30,31] In the operative management of human diabetic patients, the inhibitory effects of epidural analgesia on the beta adrenergic activity and subsequently on metabolic responses have been found to be beneficial.[13] Although propranolol inhibits the lactate, NEFA, and glucose levels in humans following gastrectomies, it has not been shown to have any deleterious effects.[7,33]

HYPOTHALAMIC–PITUITARY SYSTEM

Adrenocorticotrophic Hormone (ACTH)

Endocrine responses following injury depend on an intact nerve supply. Experimental work in dogs has demonstrated a lack of an endocrine response to injury when the part of the body traumatized had prior denervation. Sensory input into the hypothalmic–pituitary system comes from the brain stem, reticular formation, limbic system, and subcortex.[16] Endotoxins may stimulate the hypothalamus directly. The hormone released varies with the stimulus.

ACTH is released from the anterior pituitary as a result of stimulation by corticotropin releasing factor (CRF) from the hypothalamus. This in turn causes the zona fasciculata of the adrenal cortex to produce higher levels of glucocorticoids. In acute and severe trauma, higher ACTH levels may also produce aldosterone release from the zona glomerulosa. The primary result is to mobilize free fatty acids (lipolysis) which can act as an energy source, and to impair hepatic enzymes that normally inactivate cortisol. This allows larger amounts of unconjugated (active) corticosteroids to become more available even though the rate of secretion may remain constant.[12] Cortisol's effect on the metabolism of carbohydrates is to stimulate gluconeogenesis by the liver and decrease the rate of glucose utilization by the body cells.[26]

During stress, amino acids are released from extrahepatic tissues, mainly muscle, and converted into glucose. This metabolism is stimulated by the increased cortisol levels and accounts for the muscle wasting often seen in chronic stress.[23]

The presence of cortisol in adequate amounts is extremely important if the animal is to withstand the stress of surgical trauma. Patients with unrecognized adrenal insufficiency or those who become that way as a result of their condition, will not tolerate stress well unless supplemented with an exogenous corticosteroid. Adrenal insufficiency is rarely the cause of death after surgical trauma, if corticosteroids are given in adrenally compromised patients. The need for recognizing the adrenal insufficiency patient is obvious. Anorexia, muscle weakness, ECG changes consistent with hyperkalemia, dehydration, collapse, and coma are but a few of the clinical findings associated with hypoadrenocorticoidism.[26]

Cortisol decreases the inflammatory and immune responses. Sodium and water retention also occur in varying degrees, potassium being excreted by the renal tubules. It is possible that cortisol binds with specific complexes of protein in the cytoplasm and nucleus, which causes the RNA molecule to help the cell adapt to its altered environment.

The stimulation of growth hormone (GH) comes under alpha adrenergic control and results not only from surgical stress but also from hypoglycemia and increased glucagon and arginine levels.[5] Similarly to ACTH, the release of GH during the stress of surgery requires afferent input from peripheral nerves. Besides its effect on protein metabolism (causing the formation and release of somatomeclin, of peptide hepatic origin), it also has direct effects on preventing glucose uptake by peripheral tissue. GH also elevates NEFA and increases ketone formation.[5]

Thyroid stimulating hormone (TSH) is released inconsistently during surgical stress. Thyroxine (T_4) rises during operative stress, but the effect of various anesthetic agents has not been separated from this surgical trauma. This T_4 increase, however, can be abolished by epidural anesthesia. Uncertainty exists regarding the role of the thyroid gland in the response to surgical injury.[5]

Antidiuretic Hormone (ADH)

The release of ADH is controlled by carotid and atrial volume receptors and central nervous system (CNS) osmoreceptors. The production and release of ADH is increased following stimuli such as hyperosmolarity and hypovolemia due to dehydration and hemorrhage, respectively. Additional stimuli resulting in ADH release include trauma, pain, and some anesthetic agents. Any water solute distortion or blood volume reduction will stimulate ADH and it in turn will exert its effect on the renal tubules. The ADH (vasopressin) affects the renal tubules by increasing renal tubule permeability and resorption of water. The result is reduced urine volume and increased urine osmolality. Sodium is retained and extracellular water volume is restored by transcapillary refill within hours after a hemorrhagic episode.[29]

The antidiuresis that follows surgery is somewhat inappropriate, since it is activated by tissue trauma and volume reduction. The administration of hypotonic solutions or water may therefore produce hyponatremia and hypotonicity rather than merely shutting off the antidiuretic hormone production.[22]

Renin–Angiotension–Aldosterone Response

The main role of this response is to aid in the preservation of circulatory volume and therefore assist cell metabolism. This system is activated by any condition that results in an ineffective circulatory volume. In man, the first four days following a moderate form of surgical insult results in an increased urinary potassium excretion and a decreased sodium excretion.[11,21] Hyperaldosteronism in the postoperative patient is due to an increased production of aldosterone by the adrenal cortex and an impaired rate of destruction by the liver.[11,18,25]

The aldosterone secretion results primarily from the renin–angiotensin stimulus. ACTH will further enhance its secretion. Renin is secreted from the renal juxtaglomerular cells and results in the transformation of hepatic derived angiotensinogen into angiotensin I in the plasma. This substance is enzymatically converted into angiotensin II, a potent vasopressor that stimulates the adrenal cortex to secrete aldosterone. Both eventually act to maintain blood pressure, the angiotensin II by its vasoconstrictive properties and the aldosterone by causing the kidney to conserve sodium, thereby supporting the plasma volume. Besides the renin source of stimulation, increased output of aldosterone results from high ACTH levels, hyperkalemia, surgical and non-surgical trauma and hemorrhage (hypovolemia). Following the acute loss of blood, aldosterone secretion may increase thirty-fold, with increased urinary excretion of aldosterone noted as well.[23]

CARBOHYDRATE METABOLISM

Carbohydrate as an energy source is needed for DNA and RNA synthesis, formation of cellular components and the transfer of nutrients and electrolytes. The stress of surgery and anesthesia results in hyperglycemia and glycosuria. The inhibition of the pancreatic production of insulin and its peripheral activity, probably via catecholamine production, is in part the cause of the hyperglycemia.[23] Other factors contributing to an increased blood glucose include peripheral carbohydrate breakdown by the action of cortisol, the mobilization of carbohydrate by growth hormone and its antagonistic effect on insulin in the periphery, and the production of gluconeogenesis owing to the release of glucagon. Carbohydrate metabolism is most important to the animal during the initial phases of trauma.[12] Later, when the glucose demand exceeds mobilization and gluconeogenesis, the breakdown of fat and protein to produce energy will ensue.[32]

PROTEIN METABOLISM

Surgical trauma results in tissue wasting and weight loss. Although this is minimal in cases of elective surgery, it takes on added importance in those cases in which a catabolic state has existed owing to the nature of the illness. In one study in humans, preoperative weight loss was the only factor that correlated with operative mortality rates.[14]

In man, the extent of weight loss has been shown to be influenced by the patient's sex, body build, preoperative nutritional status, the degree of injury associated with the procedure, and the presence of any complicating factors such as infection.[14] Tissue loss is the result of both a nutritional deficit and neuroendocrine mechanisms activated by injury.

Following surgery, normal caloric intake is usually decreased, while catabolism is increased.[10] The intensity and duration of the postoperative catabolic period depends on the nature of the injury and whether sepsis or another major complication is present. After an elective procedure there is little effect on the expenditure of energy. However, severe fractures, or major abdominal surgery may cause a 10–30 percent increase, while sepsis and severe burns can increase energy expenditure by 60 and 200 percent, respectively.

The plasma proteins decline after injury, and this is primarily reflected in the albumin fraction.[12] It decreases after moderate injury in man by 25–30 percent on the fourth or fifth day and gradually returns to normal.[17] The return to normal depends on the extent and duration of the injury.[17] Burns depress albumin for a prolonged period of time, taking months to return to normal in some cases.[17]

Urinary nitrogen excretion increases after injury and is primarily in the form of urea nitrogen. This excretion begins soon after surgical insult and continues sometimes for weeks. The source of the urinary loss is not only from simple catabolism of body protein, but is also found to be from the synthesis of protein as well. The catabolic source of protein comes primarily from skeletal muscle with the liver and other active organs being spared. More athletic, muscular animals would presumably have a higher urinary protein loss since the major source of protein is from protein stores in the muscles. Multiple surgeries done over a short span of time usually result in less protein loss, probably due to the storage protein having been lost by the previous surgery.[12]

Since carbohydrates serve as the main source of energy following surgical trauma, protein stores are spared but eventually are converted to carbohydrates for energy through gluconeogenesis.[29] During this period of stress, any exogenous protein does not contribute to tissue repair but serves as an energy source. Only when large amounts of readily utilized calories and protein are provided during the catabolic period can the net nitrogen loss be halted.[29] This means that the metabolic effects of trauma on protein nutrition are mainly attributable to factors other than starvation. The severe stimulus for protein catabolism during the early posttrauma period is, as mentioned before, quite difficult to overcome by providing exogenous nutrients.[27] The main hormonal trigger for the catabolism of trauma is probably due to the release of catecholamines from the adrenal medulla.[29]

Following most uncomplicated surgeries, the patient will enter the catabolic phase of surgical convalescence on the third or fourth postoperative day. The anabolic steroids act on protein in an opposite way to that of the glucocorticoids. They cause protein to reenter the skeletal muscles and form connective tissue.[11] Ingested protein is retained and a positive nitrogen balance is finally achieved. Urinary nitrogen losses decrease later on to further enhance the positive nitrogen balance.

FAT METABOLISM

The importance of endogenous fat stores as sources of energy often goes unappreciated. Although tissues such as the brain, erythrocytes, and peripheral nerves are obliged to utilize glucose as their sole energy source, other tissues can catabolize fatty acids and their metabolic products (ketones) and use them for energy.[29] This occurs as carbohydrate availability becomes diminished.

During starvation, increasing amounts of fatty acids derived from body fat can provide an energy source by conversion into acetylcoenzyme A and participate in the tricarboxylic acid cycle. By-products of this shift in metabolic pathways are excreted in the urine, and when these substances are produced in excess, a state of ketoacidosis may exist.[11]

The increase in plasma unesterified fatty acids normally seen soon after a surgical episode, can be counteracted by the injection of glucose.[11,33] Fatty metabolism can also be markedly decreased by early resumption of food intake after surgery. When fats again start being stored, the patient enters the fat gain phase of convalescence. Fat is stored in adipose tissue mostly as triglycerides to become readily available again as an energy source.[11] The fat gain phase lasts for several weeks after a moderately severe surgical procedure or longer following more severe surgical trauma.[11]

FLUID AND ELECTROLYTE SHIFTS

In the injured animal several mechanisms act to conserve extracellular fluid and maintain blood volume.[29] The volume of extracellular fluid has a higher biologic priority than the maintenance of its precise chemical composition.[22] Sodium conservation is the key, with renal retention of water being important as well. The fluid conserving mechanism (ADH) causes a sharp restriction in the excretion of free water. Urine osmolality is seen to rise owing to distal tubular resorbtion.[22] Combined with fluid therapy during and after surgery, dilutional hyponatremia is often the result. This occurs in spite of the sodium retention caused by the release of aldosterone in response to a surgical anesthetic episode.[20] The angiotensin secreted during this response will cause some degree of vasoconstriction and subsequently decrease the glomerular filtration rate (GFR). These effects last only a few days, especially if the condition is uncomplicated by major and severe surgery, prolonged anesthesia, infections, and severe hemorrhage.

The ADH secretion is capable of being suppressed to varying degrees by maintaining good hydration preoperatively and during anesthesia. Little effect on ADH secretion is accomplished during a major operation or in the postoperative period. The water retention, oliguria and hyponatremia are changes compounded by giving solute free fluids and to a minor degree by water released during the oxidation of fat.[12]

Potassium is lost via renal excretion in relatively large quantities post-injury. This loss is promoted by aldosterone and cortisol. The potassium stored with glycogen is released during glycogenolysis and from severely damaged tissues. Acidosis will drive potassium from the cell while alkalosis will drive it intracellularly.

The phosphate anion rises immediately after a prolonged operation and reflects a decrease in GFR. It also is released from muscle and liver.

The hydrogen ion (HI) will usually increase in concentration (acidosis) as the magnitude of the injury increases. Shock and renal failure will contribute greatly to an acidotic state. The elevated HI concentration is also associated with a release of organic and inorganic acids. Acids contributing to a lower pH include lactate, fatty acids, ketones, phosphate and sulfate. The lactate ion increases greatly when tissues are poorly perfused with blood.

RENAL RESPONSE TO INJURY

The risk of irreversible renal damage following surgery is greatest if there is any degree of renal disease prior to surgery and anesthesia. The kidney is easily insulted because it is the target organ for the interplay of a wide variety of influences following trauma. The mechanism that triggers water or sodium retention may at the same time have a deleterious effect on the kidney. Differential renal vasoconstriction is a response to any blood volume or flow challenge.[23]

Extrinsic causes of oliguria include such things as external fluid loss, hemorrhage, dehydration, gastrointestinal fluid loss, or internal "third space" accumulation of fluid as seen with bowel obstruction, gastric dilation–volvulus complex, pancreatitis, peritonitis, or limb trauma.[23]

Intrinsic renal damage causing oliguria is due to acute tubular necrosis.[2] This results from renal vasoconstriction coupled with shunting of blood away from the renal cortex, decreased filtration fraction of renal blood flow and a maximal resorptive stimulus by aldosterone and ADH.[23] Adequate hydration and solute loading help protect the kidney from these normal responses to surgical trauma.

RESPIRATORY DISEASE AND ITS EFFECTS ON THE SURGICAL PATIENT

Because of the increased morbidity and mortality in patients going to surgery with lung disease, it is mandatory that the risks of surgery be given prime consideration. The risks depend on the clinical status of the animal and the type of surgery that will be performed. One can anticipate a more unfavorable outcome in pulmonary cripples if thoracic surgery is done, compared to a minor nonthoracic procedure.

Alterations of pulmonary function after all kinds of surgical trauma are common and can potentially develop into a postoperative pulmonary complication in previously normal patients. Prophylactic measures taken in higher-risk patients can insure a better outcome.[34]

Pulmonary abnormalities following surgery are due to a composite of events to which patients are exposed during the perioperative period. These include the surgical procedure itself, anesthesia, restrictive bandages, sensorium changes, postoperative medications (specifically analgesics), and lateral recumbency on one side for a prolonged period of time.[32] There are four areas in which these events can exert an influence: (1) lung volumes, (2) pattern of ventilation, (3) gas exchange (4) defense mechanisms.[30]

Total lung capacity and its subdivisions are often affected, especially if abdominal or thoracic surgery is performed.[30] In one human study non-abdominal, nonthoracic surgery did not affect vital capacity whereas abdominal surgery decreased the vital capacity by 25–50 percent.[1,3,4,6,7] Decreased functional residual capacity is an added problem in our animal patients if the thorax has been surgically invaded and a pleural filling defect (pneumothorax, hemothorax) remains postoperatively (see Ch. 6).

Surgery often affects the pattern of ventilation as well as the work of breathing, the degree of which depends on the nature of the surgical injury. Tidal volume is severely affected in thoracic surgical procedures where pain and discomfort play an important role in preventing good chest excursion. The fall in tidal volume may be due to a decrease in lung compliance. Elastic work required to inflate the lung goes up as the square of the increase in tidal volume.[24] Tachypnea combined with shallow breathing can severely decrease tidal volume to the point of hypoxia and hypercarbia in the postoperative period.

The importance of good ventilation under anesthesia is underscored by several studies in dogs demonstrating a clear cut decrease in compliance if periodic hyperinflation was not performed.[19,32] Functional residual capacity was also decreased in these dogs.[9,19] This decrease in compliance was noted during postmortem examination to be due at least in part to airway closure.[9] This appeared to be most severe in the dependent portions of the lungs.

A gas exchange problem in animals postoperatively is often seen.[8] The decrease in PaO_2 is thought to be directly related to the effects of positioning, lack of turning and the type of surgery on the ventilation–perfusion (V/Q) ratio. Studies in rabbits undergoing thoracotomies reveal an increase in venous admixture thought to be produced by perfusion of collapsed alveoli.[27] More severe lung disease in thoracic surgery patients could result in retention of carbon dioxide as well a more severe gas exchange problem.

The cough mechanism is an important defense against secretion and particulate matter that tend to deposit in the upper airways during a surgical and anesthetic experience. Clearance from lower airways depends on maintaining the integrity of the mucociliary system, the alveoli, the cellular components, and lymphatic drainage.[32] Tracheobronchial secretions and their evacuation are of prime importance if the normal defense mechanisms of the pulmonary tree are to be preserved.

A variety of factors posttrauma can threaten the integrity of the lungs. Airway compromise may result due to aspiration of gastric contents or prolonged positional immobilization. Some other factors include such things as fluid overload with oncotic dilution and pulmonary edema, and underlying heart failure. Vasoactive substances affecting pulmonary perfusion can contribute to pulmonary compromise, especially serotonin from platelets, catecholamines and the kinins.[23] Chest wall mechanics threaten lung integrity and can be due to an unstable rib cage or sternum following closure of the chest wound. If open chest surgery is prolonged, collapsed or underperfused lungs can also be a factor contributing to pulmonary dysfunction.

Those prophylactic measures recommended to decrease postoperative complications would include intraoperative considerations such as: decreased length of anesthesia, evacuation of secretions, prevention of aspiration, and intermittent hyperinflation. Postoperative measures would include the continuation of hyperinflation, good tracheobronchial toiletry, early ambulation, no antitussive medication, and analgesics to control pain with special emphasis on monitoring the effects of the analgesic on the pattern of breathing.[32]

CARDIAC FUNCTION OF THE PATIENT UNDERGOING SURGICAL TRAUMA

The surgical metabolism and ability of the patient to withstand surgical trauma depends greatly on good cardiovascular function. This organ is a "flow sensitive organ" as are the brain and kidneys.[23] It is one of the organs that should be evaluated closely when subjecting the patient to any form of surgical trauma.

Many factors during surgery and anesthesia are potentially deleterious to good cardiac function. These include acidosis, hypoxemia, hypercapnia, decreased systemic vascular resistance, decreased myocardial contractility, and hypotension due to hypovolemia or other nonvolume-related factors. Dysrhythmias due to catecholamine release, bradycardia associated with some muscle relaxants (succinylcholine), and decreased coronary flow due to a diminished systemic flow are additional cardiac hazards.

Although cardiac output decreases intraoperatively due to a decrease in stroke volume in man,[12] an elevated cardiac output postoperatively is the normal response.[23] This is thought to be due to the catecholamine influence and a shift leftward of the hemoglobin dissociation curve in those patients who have been hyperventilated during surgery or which have hypocarbia due to hyperventilation secondary to pain, stress, and anxiety.[23] Massive blood transfusions can cause a deficiency in 2,3 DPG and complement the effect of respiratory acidosis on the oxyhemoglobin dissociation curve. Because of the decreased oxygen extraction by the tissues, cardiac output is increased by a compensatory mechanism working to correct a disorder of oxygen transport. Some patients with other underlying pathology such as lactic acidosis, congestive heart failure, cardiac dysrhythmias or renal failure may not accept this challenge of increased cardiac output and must be cautiously monitored postoperatively. The heart is also affected by the nutritional status of the patients as proposed by some investigators who have shown adverse effects on the hearts of rats maintained in a protein deficient state.[15]

THE GASTROINTESTINAL SYSTEM AND THE SURGICAL PATIENT

Following surgical trauma, the stomach usually shows decreased motility and delayed emptying. The increased sympathetic influence is responsible for most of this effect. With severe trauma, achlorhydria may be present.[16]

The secretions of the intestine are usually unaffected, but motility and absorption of fluids are decreased, sometimes to the point of gastrointestinal "pooling" of fluid. During recovery, motility usually returns before absorption, and as a result the stools may be watery.

SURGICAL CONVALESCENCE

Barring unforeseen complications, there is usually a shorter catabolic phase and a longer anabolic phase following a surgical procedure. The four phases associated with the postoperative course of recovery have been described as: (1) injury (catabolic) phase, (2) turning point (equilibrium), (3) anabolic phase, and (4) fat gain.[21,23]

The catabolic phase can be influenced by the knowledge and skill of the surgeon, as the depth and duration of the injury during the surgical procedure can be diminished in many cases. Minimal trauma to tissues, accurate restoration of fluid volumes, careful placement of sutures and adequate immobilization of bone injuries, will all work to minimize the pain, the degree of endocrine response and the total stimulus of injury.[23]

The turning point phase is the most dramatic period. The animal will return to normal eating, ambulation, eliminations and will display behavior most often seen in a better state of health (e.g., grooming as seen in cats).

The anabolic phase is characterized by an increase in strength, further increase in appetite and ambulation, and the maintenance of a positive nitrogen balance until the preinjury levels have been restored.[23]

The fat gain phase follows the return of nitrogen metabolism to zero balance. Any caloric intake that exceeds the zero balance will now result in the deposition of body fat and further weight gain. This weight gain may be a problem in some animals, especially those that are immobilized and have a decrease in activity due to their surgical illness, must notably, neurosurgical or orthopedic patients. Some degree of dietary restraint may be necessary if normal activity and exercise cannot be regained after post injury anabolism is complete.[22]

HEMATOLOGIC AND BLOOD CHEMISTRY VALUES IN RESPONSE TO SURGICAL STRESS

The surgeon should be aware of how surgical trauma will affect hematologic and biochemical parameters. This enhances the ability to discern real complications from normal postoperative alterations. A more rational approach to treatment versus no treatment is gained from this knowledge. Major surgery causes a greater change in mean values than minor surgery in all but one of the parameters elevated in a recent study.[28]

The white blood count (WBC) mean changes from 6.8 ($\cdot 10^3$/mm^3) preop to the highest mean at 24 hours postop (16.98). Neutrophilia combined with a lymphopenia and eosinopenia occur consistently. Blood urea nitrogen (BUN) values elevate significantly from the preoperative value and remain so for 2 weeks.

Other significant values that are elevated from preoperative or immediate postop values (24–48 hours) include alkaline phosphatase, total bilirubin, serum cortisol and creatinine. Elevated cortisol levels are anticipated and appear to correlate well with minor versus major surgical trauma, being significantly higher with the latter.[28]

REFERENCES

1. Anscombe AR, Buxton RS: Effect of abdominal operations on total lung capacity and its subdivisions. Br Med J 2:84, 1958
2. Arieff AI, Forshan PH, Sokolow M et al: Special medical problems in surgical patients. In Dunphy JE Way LW (eds): Current Surgical Diagnosis and Treatment. 3rd Ed. Lange, Los Altos, 1977
3. Beecher HK: The measured effect of laparotomy on respiration. J Clin Invest 12:639, 1933
4. Beecher HK: Effect of laparotomy on lung volume: demonstration of a new type of pulmonary collapse. J Clin Invest 12:651, 1933
5. Burke JF: Surgical Physiology. WB Saunders, Philadelphia, 1983
6. Churchill ED, McNeil D: The reduction in vital capacity following operation. Surg Gynecol Obstet 44:483, 1927
7. Cooper GM, Paterson JL, Mashiter K et al: Beta adrenergic blockade and the metabolic response to surgery. Br J Anaesth 52:1231, 1980
8. Diament ML, Palmer KNV: Postoperative changes in gas tensions of arterial blood and in ventilatory function. Lancet 2:180, 1966
9. Dubois AB, Botelho SY, Bedell GN et al: A rapid plethysmographic method for measuring thoracic gas volume: comparison with a nitrogen washout method for measuring functional residual capacity in normals. J Clin Invest 35:322, 1956
10. Elwyn DH, Kinney JM, Askanazi J: Energy expenditure in surgical patients. Surg Clin North Am 61:545, 1981
11. Henegar GC: Metabolic and endocrine effects of injury and surgery. In Preston FW and Beal JM (eds): Basic Surgical Physiology. Yearbook Medical Publishers, Chicago, 1969
12. Hume DM: Endocrine and metabolic responses to injury. In Schwarz S (ed): Principles of Surgery. 2nd Ed. McGraw-Hill, New York, 1974
13. Kehlet H, Brandt MR, Hansen AP et al: Effect of epidural anesthesia on metabolic profiles during and after surgery. Br J Surg 66:543, 1979
14. Kinney JM, Long CL, Gump FE et al: Tissue composition of weight loss in surgical patients, I. Elective operation. Ann Surg 168:459, 1968
15. Kyger ER, Block WJ, Roach G et al: Adverse effects of protein malnutrition on myocardial function. Surgery 84:147, 1978

16. Lantz G: Small animal surgery course outline. Purdue University, West Lafayette, IN, 1981
17. Ledingham IM, Mackay C, Jamieson RA, Kay, AW: Metabolic response to injury. In Jamieson & Kay (eds): Textbook of Surgical Physiology. 3rd Ed. Churchill Livingstone, New York, 1978
18. Llaurado JG, Woodruff MFA: Postoperative transient aldosteronism. Surgery 42:313, 1957
19. Mead J, Collier C: Relation of volume history of lungs to respiratory mechanics in dogs. J Appl Physiol 14:669, 1959
20. Michell AR: The metabolic consequences of trauma. J Small Anim Pract 15:279, 1974
21. Moore, FD: Bodily changes in surgical convalescence I; normal sequence-observations and interpretations. Ann Surg 137:289, 1953
22. Moore FD: Metabolic Care of The Surgical Patient. WB Saunders, Philadelphia, 1959
23. Moore FD: Homeostasis: Bodily changes in trauma and surgery. In Sabiston DC, Jr (ed): Text Book of Surgery. WB Saunders, Philadelphia, 1972
24. Peters RM, Wellons HA, Htwe, TM et al: Total compliance and work of breathing after thoracotomy. J Thorac Cardiovasc Surg 57:348, 1969
25. Riveron E, Kukral JC, Henegar GC: Blood volume, water, and electrolyte spaces in human beings with cirrhosis and in dogs with Eck's fistula. Surg Forum 17:365, 1966
26. Rosin E: The systemic response to injury. In Bojrab MJ (ed): Pathophysiology in Small Animal Surgery. Lea & Febiger, Philadelphia, 1981
27. Sackur: Zur lehre vom pneumothorax. Zentralblatt fur Klinical Medizine 29:1896
28. Schmid RE, Booker JL: Effects of different surgical stresses on hematologic and blood chemistry values in dogs. J Am Vet Assoc Sept/Oct: 758, 1982
29. Sheldon GF, Harper HA, Way LW: In Dunphy JE, Way LW (eds): Current Surgical Diagnosis and Treatment. 3rd Ed. Lange, Los Altos, 1977
30. Snow PJD: Treatment of acute myocardial injection with propranolol. Am J Cardiol 18:458, 1966
31. Sokolow M, Forshan PH, Wilson JL et al: Special medical problems in surgical patients. In Dunphy JE, Way LW (eds): Current Surgical Diagnosis and Treatment. 3rd Ed. Lange, Los Altos, 1977
32. Tisi GM: State of the art preoperative evaluation of pulmonary function. Am Rev Respir Dis 119:293, 1979
33. Tsuji H, Asoh T, Shirasaica C et al: Inhibition of metabolic response to surgery with beta adrenergic blockade. Br J Surg 67:503, 1980
34. Wigton DH, Kociba GJ, Wilson G: Alterations of specific hematologic parameters in normal dogs due to surgical stress. (abstract) Arch Am Coll Vet Surg 4:3, 1975
35. Wilson JL: Respiratory disease in the surgical patient. In Dunphy JE, Way LW (eds): Current Surgical Diagnosis and Treatment. 3rd Ed. Lange, Los Altos, 1977

2 | Intravenous Therapy and Blood Transfusion

Marc R. Raffe

Fluid therapy and blood replacement may be critical to short- and long-term survival of the emergency surgical candidate. In many cases, deficits in fluid, electrolyte, or blood components are intensified by the metabolic response to injury and contemporary loss from the injury site. Restoration of deficits allows for reestablishment of circulatory stability and overall fluid balance. The decisions the clinician is burdened with are what type of fluid, colloid, or blood component should be used, the quantity to be administered, and the ideal composition of the replacement therapy. The goals of this chapter are to provide background information concerning fluid composition and choice, to formulate therapeutic guidelines, and to outline potential complications intrinsic to the administration of replacement therapy.

CRYSTALLOID THERAPY

Indications for Therapy

General indications for crystalloid therapy include replacement of contemporary fluid loss, restoration of preexisting fluid deficits, and provision for anticipated fluid requirements that will not be met by normal routes of fluid intake. One or more of these categories are present in any surgical candidate. In the routine surgical patient, preoperative water volume deficits can be anticipated if water and food are withheld for eight to twelve hours. An insensible water loss of at least 2 ml/kg/hr will occur in the intervening time.[17]

In the emergency surgical candidate, additional routes of preoperative water loss may include external wounds, gastrointestinal losses, tissue sequestration from shock, and frank blood loss. Compensatory mechanisms may lead to an isotonic transfer of fluid from functional to nonfunctional body compartments. This type of extracellular (ECF) volume deficit is defined as a distribution disturbance. This fluid sequestration is maintained in the interstitial water compartment, which does not contribute to vascular water balance. With an increased interstitial fluid component, a relative dessication of intravascular plasma volume occurs. This compartmental shift renders the animal susceptible to hypotension and the development of oliguria. These deficiencies are exacerbated by subsequent exposure to anesthetic agents that may further accentuate fluid deficits through direct effects on cardiovascular perfusion, renal blood flow, and attenuation of autonomic nervous system tone. Resolution of fluid sequestration occurs with time. In man, the period of resolution occurs in the course of one to three post-injury days. Most fluid liberated from sequestered sites exits the body as urine.[13,16,17]

Evaluation of Fluid Status

Proper fluid and electrolyte support depends on careful physical and clinicopathologic data evaluation during the preoperative period. Sources of information may include mental status, water consumption history, heart rate, pulse quality, skin turgor, mucous membrane moisture and urine output. Laboratory data may include packed cell volume (PCV), total solids, osmolality, serum sodium, potassium, and chloride levels, blood urea nitrogen content (BUN), and acid-base evaluation. By analyzing this data, evaluation of volume, concentration, and composition of replacement fluid may be obtained. Perioperative evaluation of fluid status includes similar measured parameters. In addition, evaluation of blood pressure, heart rate, heart sounds, and electrocardiographic monitoring may all contribute to evaluation of fluid balance. Measurement of volume loss from surgical suction and estimation of surgical sponge content may provide additional data. Reevaluation of baseline laboratory parameters listed above may provide further information. Urine production may also be collected and measured. The dynamics of the perioperative period demand constant reevaluation and adjustment of therapy to maintain support. Continuous monitoring of volume loss is the critical factor and appropriate replacement therapy is administered to correct deficits. In addition to volume loss, compositional and concentration losses must also be evaluated. Loss of sodium, potassium, and chloride, plus evaluation of acid-base balance is critical in replacement therapy during this time.[16,17]

Postoperative fluid therapy should be continued to reverse deficits remaining from the pre- and perioperative periods and for replacement of contemporary and maintenance fluid requirements until water and salt balance can be reestablished. A continuation of the principles used in the perioperative period should occur such that changing trends in requirements can be monitored and corrected as they occur.[16,17]

Types of Intravenous Fluids

Crystalloid fluids may be subcategorized into maintenance, replacement, or special purpose groups. Maintenance fluids generally are designed to provide replacement for insensible fluid losses, which generally are sodium free. Routes of loss include pulmonary tract, stool, and urine in domestic species. Because these losses are essentially sodium free, maintenance solutions are hypotonic with respect to sodium. Examples include five percent dextrose in water, 0.45 percent sodium chloride, and hypotonic polyionic solutions (Normosol-M, Plasmalyte 56).[16,17]

Replacement fluids are formulated to approximate extracellular fluid composition. Selection of replacement fluids generally incorporates replacement of losses from interstitial edema, gastric or fistula drainage, pleural or ascitic fluid, and wound sites. Replacement fluids should have sodium concentrations approximating extracellular fluid. Examples of replacement fluid include lactated Ringer's, Hartmann's solution and Normosol-R. Additional preparations are noted in Table 2-1.[16,17]

Special purpose fluids are formulated for specific fluid and electrolyte therapy. Hypertonic bicarbonate solution (8.4 percent) and hypertonic saline (3 percent) are two examples of this class. Special purpose fluids are formulated or indicated for specific disturbances in electrolyte or acid-base balance which may not be corrected by conventional solution therapy or must be administered under limited volume (water restriction).[16,17]

Intraoperative Fluid Administration

A plethora of "routines" for intraoperative fluid therapy exist, many based on little scientific data. A spectrum of support from no fluid support to massive quantity infusion is present in veterinary medicine. The concept to appreciate is that no *ideal value* exists, and that fluid therapy must be appropriately administered to each animal. The following is a prudent plan for fluid administration during the perioperative period. Recognize that a base assumption of no preexisting deficits in fluid, electrolyte, or acid-base status are presnt. Deficit calculations will be subsequently presented.

Many animals are fasted for a variable time prior to anesthetic induction. If water is withheld during this time (6–8 hours), then a negative water balance exists in the anesthesia candidate. In general, a value of 2 ml/kg/hr may be used to calculate insensible water loss during this period. This volume should be replaced in the first 40 to 45 minutes of the anesthetic period. From this point, the surgery should be classified as a maintenance or replacement type of procedure. Maintenance procedures are those in which minimal fluid or blood loss is anticipated. Maintenance composition fluids are selected in these cases and infused at a rate to replace insensible loss, correct for preoperative dessication, and provide volume expansion to compensate for altered vascular compliance from anesthetic agents. In general, 2–4 ml/kg/hr is adequate for this purpose.[16,17]

Table 2-1. Commercially Available Fluids for Intravenous Use

Solution	Type	Carbohydrate (mg/ml)	Sodium (mEq/L)	Other Cations	Chloride (mEq/L)	Other Anions (mEq/L)
5% Dextrose	M[a]	50	—	—	—	—
5% Dextrose with 0.45% NaCl	M	50	77	—	77	—
Normosol-M (5% Dextrose)	M	0 (50)	40	K13[b], Mg3[c]	40	Acetate (16)
Plasmalyte 56 (5% Dextrose)	M	0 (50)		K13, Mg3	140	Acetate (16)
Ringer's (2.5, 5% Dextrose)	R[d]	0 (25, 50)	40	K4, Ca5[e]	156	—
Lactated Ringer's (2.5, 5% Dextrose)	R	0 (25, 50)	130	K4, Ca3	109	Lactate (28)
Hartmann's (5% Dextrose)	R	0 (50)	131	K4, Ca4	111	Lactate (27)
Normosol-R (5% Dextrose)	R	0 (50)	140	K4, Mg3	98	Acetate, Gluconate (50)
Plasmalyte 148 (5% Dextrose)	R	0 (50)	140	K10, Ca5, Mg3	103	Acetate, Lactate (55)
0.9% NaCl (5% Dextrose)	R	0 (50)	154	—	154	—
5% NaCl	SP[f]	—	855	—	855	—
NaHCO₃ (8.4%)	SP	—	1,000	—	—	Bicarbonate (1,000)

[a] M = Maintenance.
[b] K = Potassium (mEq/L).
[c] Mg = Magnesium (mEq/L).
[d] R = Replacement.
[e] Ca = Calcium (mEq/L).
[f] SP = Special Procedure.

Table 2-2. Guidelines for Perioperative Fluid Support

A. Maintenance Fluid Requirement
   1. Replace insensible losses with a maintenance composition fluid at 2–4 ml/kg/hr since cessation of oral water ingestion.
B. Replacement Fluid Requirement
   1. Add a replacement solution for intraoperative insensible fluid losses at 2 ml/kg/hr.
   2. Add according to degree of surgical trauma:
      Minimal—4 ml/kg/hr
      Moderate—6 ml/kg/hr
      Severe—8 ml/kg/hr
   3. Add colloid solution if blood volume loss is greater than 20 percent.
C. Deficit Fluid Requirement
   1. Add replacement solution at rate to provide deficit replacement calculated on an hourly basis. Calculate deficit requirement by standard formulae.
D. Contemporary Fluid Requirement
   1. Add replacement solution, colloids, or blood components as needed to replenish contemporary loss other than surgical trauma.

Adapted from Gieseke AH: Perioperative Fluid Therapy. In Miller RD (ed): Anesthesia, Churchill Livingstone, New York, 1981.

If a significant loss of blood or fluid is anticipated in the perioperative period, then a replacement procedure is followed. A balanced, polyionic replacement fluid is selected for use. The anticipated degree of surgical trauma and blood loss is factored into replacement infusion rates. If minimal surgical trauma is anticipated, the animal should receive 2 ml/kg/hr for nonsurgical fluid requirements plus 4 ml/kg/hr for surgical trauma. The infusion of 6 ml/kg/hr is composed of polyionic solutions such as lactated Ringer's solution or Normosol-R. Moderate surgical trauma is anticipated in surgical procedures invading body cavities or superficial limb tissue. These cases require 2 ml/kg/hr plus 6 ml/kg/hr for moderate trauma, or a total of 8 ml/kg/hr. Extensive surgical trauma requires aggressive fluid therapy management. Fracture repair, bowel obstruction, extensive reconstructive surgery, and other traumatic procedures require 2 ml/kg/hr plus 8 ml/kg/hr for surgical trauma, or a total of 10 mg/kg/hr[17] (Table 2-2).

Monitoring the response to fluid therapy is important. Heart rate, pulse quality, heart sounds, and blood pressure may all be evaluated for fluid therapy response. Urine output is a good overall indicator of fluid therapy response. Central venous pressure (CVP) provides data about right ventricular response to fluid administration, but is not a direct measure of fluid replacement adequacy. Definitive information is obtained by the use of pulmonary artery catheterization and cardiac output measurement.[16,17]

If preexisting deficits in fluid balance exist, then an additional consideration of deficit correction must occur during the perioperative period. In addition to anticipated requirements listed above (2 ml/kg/hr insensible loss plus contemporary surgical site loss), inclusion of an additional quantity for preexisting deficits must be calculated. From clinical evaluation, calculation of total fluid deficit in the animal can be performed. Using standard procedure, a 75 percent correction of deficit should occur during the initial 24-hour period, with the remaining 25 percent correction occurring by 48 hours. If surgery is performed during this time, then the hourly deficit replacement is added to contemporary losses. For example, if a 240 ml deficit is calculated for an animal, then 10 ml/hr is infused as a deficit replacement during surgery. Do not administer the entire deficit volume during the perioperative period. Equilibration between water compartments will not occur and ECF overload may produce interstitial tissue edema in previously debilitated animals. The assumption that adequate renal function safeguards the patient from volume or salt excess is invalid. Alteration in water and salt modulation occurs during general anesthesia. Reduction in glomerular filtration rate, elevation in antidiuretic hormone and renin levels, and increased renal vascular resistance contribute to decreased urine production. Polyionic solutions may attenuate this response, however, and baseline function may not be present in all cases.[13,16,17]

Concepts related to crystalloid infusion change dramatically in the intensive care environment. Acute decompensation of hemodynamic function can occur as a result of blood loss and shock. Stabilization by volume expansion to restore circulating blood volume is mandatory during this time. Crystalloid fluid infusion is a valuable method of volume replacement. Rapid infusion of up to 90 ml/kg/hr is tolerated in healthy dogs with a wide safely margin. A general guideline of a 3 : 1 replacement ratio of crystalloid : blood loss has been described to account for ultimate compartmental redistribution. Administration usually is continued until therapeutic response is observed. Mucous membrane color improvement, restoration of urine production, decreased heart rate, and improved pulse character all indicate response to therapy. Quantitative measurement of blood pressure, central venous pressure, and pulmonary artery pressure provide additional information.[11,40]

Complications

Most complications attributed to crystalloids are not a result of their use per se, but reflect misjudgments or the errors in technique of administration. Major objections to the use of large-volume resuscitation with crystalloid fluid have been debated for several decades. Issues regarding hemodilution, development of pulmonary edema, and administration of exogenous lactate have been raised regarding crystalloid resuscitation during shock and hemorrhagic states. None of these objections have been substantiated with crystalloid administration. Hemodilution of erythrocyte mass theoretically lowers the oxygen carrying capacity of the blood. The clinical significance of this is equivocal as hemodilution actually improves oxygen transport until packed cell volume approaches 25 percent. This improvement is a reflection of improved cardiac output and microcirculation resulting from lowered blood viscosity. No increase in incidence of hemostatic defects can be attributed to hemodilution.[40]

Pulmonary edema has been a critical issue in the use of high-volume crystalloid resuscitation. Dilution of intravascular colloid components may reduce vascular oncotic pressure. Fluid movement into the interstitial compartment and development of tissue edema may result. This theoretical disadvantage has not been proven in several well-controlled studies in animals and people. Acute hemodynamic resuscitation using crystalloids until colloid or blood components were available produced no significant increase in development of pulmonary edema, when compared to cases resuscitated only with colloid or blood products. In several studies, pulmonary complications increased with use of albumin or synthetic colloids, when compared to crystalloid infusion. In preexisting respiratory distress syndrome, colloid or blood administration improved oxygen transport when compared to crystalloid infusion during early disease course. However, no benefit was noted during terminal periods. Pulmonary edema can be induced by gross overadministration of crystalloid volume. Pulmonary tissue response would differ little from other tissue systems in this circumstance. In healthy dogs without preexisting cardiovascular disease, infusion rates up to 225 ml/kg/hr can be tolerated during a short resuscitation period (one hour) with only transient changes in hemodynamic parameters. Clinical signs of chemosis and nasal discharge are the only signs referable to massive infusion rate.[11,17]

Lactic acidemia is an anticipated sequela of the shock cycle. Although concern has been expressed over administration of exogenous lactate to patients with elevated endogenous lactate levels, no evidence exists to support exclusion of lactated Ringer's solution during therapy. Ringer's lactate has not been shown to contribute to the excess lactate levels accompanying shock. Improvement of circulatory dynamics and restoration of microcirculation restores hepatic perfusion and oxygen delivery. Exogenous and endogenous lactate is then hepatically biotransformed to bicarbonate, which aids in restoration of buffer base balance.[17,40]

Fluid temperature may affect cardiovascular resuscitation. Ringer's lactate at 40°F, 75°F, and 98.6°F was administered to dogs at rates approximating resuscitation volumes (50 ml per minute). Adverse effects on heart rate, blood pressure, electrocardiographic rhythm, and survival were noted with infusion of cold (40°F) solutions. Room temperature (75°F) and heated (98.6°F) fluids were well tolerated with only a slight change in electrocardiographic appearance noted in the group given solutions at room temperature.[10]

COLLOID SOLUTIONS

Colloids are substances that are not freely permeable to vascular endothelium owing to molecular size or structure. Their presence, based on the Starling equation and principles governing solute balance (Donnan-Gibbs equation) exerts osmotic pressure for retention of free water in the intravascular space. Colloid substances generally considered for use include fractioned albumin, low- and high-molecular-weight dextrans, hydroxyethyl starch preparations, and whole or fractionated blood components.[14,18]

Indications for Use

Colloids have been advocated for use on the basis of greater stability of circulating vascular volume and a lower incidence of postresuscitation edema in the interstitial compartment. Their use is primarily advocated for the treatment of hypovolemia and shock. Composition of colloids dictates their effective duration of activity and the degree of oncotic pressure exerted in the plasma compartment. In general, synthetic colloids represented by dextrans and starch preparations exert a shorter duration of effect prior to elimination from the vascular space. Their effective duration of activity ranges from 2 hours for low-molecular-weight dextrans (Dextran 40) to 6 hours for hydroxyethyl starch and high-molecular-weight dextrans (Dextran 60–75). Albumin exhibits a longer duration of activity, ranging from 4 to 15 days[14] (Table 2-3).

Advantages of Colloid Administration

Use of colloids diminishes the crystalloid volume replacement necessary during vascular resuscitation. They may be used on an equivolume basis for replacement of vascular volume loss. Their activity in maintaining intravascular oncotic pressure has proven valuable in combination with crystalloid infusion to maintain fluid balance between the vascular and interstitial compartments. The antithrombogenic effect and maintenance of microcirculation attributed to colloid administration are beneficial during the acute resuscitation period. Improvement in microcirculation and oxygen delivery has been shown in hypovolemic or septic shock. Provision of vascular compartment stability during chronic disease states also favors use of colloid replacement therapy. Albumin remains the first choice in this application.[14,17,37]

Disadvantages of Colloid Therapy

The benefits of colloid therapy are controversial in many cases. Acute vascular resuscitation is satisfactorily performed using crystalloid products. Inclusion of colloids in the resuscitation period has been shown to improve intravascular water retention; however, duration of benefit is brief with most products. Valuable effects on pulmonary function have been documented with colloid administration. Most studies evaluating naturally occurring cardiovascular trauma indicate mixed results from the administration of colloids when oxygen uptake and transport were measured. Early periods of respiratory distress syndrome in man have been shown to benefit from colloid use; no advantage was noted later in the disease course. In man, colloid-associated pulmonary dysfunction has been reported. Newer synthetic colloids represented by hydroxyethyl starch appear to exhibit a lower incidence of pulmonary complications. Analogous studies are currently unavailable in domestic species.[17,32,37]

Incompatibility reactions have been documented with colloid administration. Gelatin base colloids have been shown to result in histamine release in dogs and people. Hypotension has accompanied administration of dextrans, gelatin, and hydroethyl starch in experimental dog studies. This was associated with histamine release with gelatin base preparations, however, no increased levels of histamine could be demonstrated with other colloid preparations. Anaphylactoid reactions have been described in man with the use of dextrans,

Table 2-3. Comparison of Colloidal Plasma Substitutes

Substitute	Production	Mean Molecular Weight	Intravascular Life Span	Immune Reaction	Severity
Plasma Protein	Blood separation	Variable (50,000)	4–15 days	Allergic	Mild–Severe
Dextran	Leuconostoc Mesentoides (B512)	40,000 or 75,000	2 hours	Antidextran antibodies Complement fixation	Mild–Severe
Starch	Acid hydrolysis treatment of soya and corn–ethylene oxide	450,000	6 hours	Complement activation	Immediate–Severe
Gelatin	Hydrolysis of animal collagens	35,000	2–3 hours	Histamine release	Immediate–Severe

Adapted from: Doenicke A, Girote B, Lorenz W: Blood and blood substitutes. Br J Anaesth 49:681, 1977.

gelatins, and hydroxyethyl starch. Clinical signs ranging from fever and erythema of the skin to complete cardiopulmonary collapse have been reported. The mechanism of reaction differs among preparations. Direct protein allergy, anticolloid antibodies, complement activation, and histamine release have been documented as reaction mechanisms.[14]

Inhibition of clot formation has been documented with dextran infusion. Reports of hemorrhagic diathesis following dextran administration has been described with long-term (greater than 24 hours) administration of high-molecular-weight dextran (Dextran 70). The clotting defects are attributed to reduction in platelet adhesiveness secondary to an antithrombin effect.[23]

A major area of concern with colloid use has been perivascular leakage of colloids through injured vessels, with development of interstitial edema. Toxic injury to endothelium or interactions from sepsis and shock have been reported to increase vascular permeability to water and colloid substances. The major concern related to transcompartmental shifts in water and colloids is the development of pulmonary edema in the postresuscitation period. This question has been debated with a variety of conclusions based upon specific circumstances. The cause and effect relationship of perfusion, tissue oxygenation, and capillary leakage is complex and directly affects experimental evidence. Most authors agree at this time that interaction of these factors must be present for pulmonary edema to develop. Aggressive administration of crystalloid solutions have been shown to increase pulmonary water content; however, this trend was reversed within 24 hours postresuscitation in animals with functional lymphatic circulation. Colloid administration can either contribute to or inhibit development of pulmonary edema, depending upon preexisting balance between factors described in the Starling equation. Elevation in left atrial pressure enhances development of pulmonary edema. Therefore, hemodynamic function during resuscitation may be a critical factor, in addition to increased capillary permeability. The integrity and function of pulmonary lymphatics in the clearance of interstitial water and albumin must also be considered. The contribution of colloids to edema formation, therefore, is a complex, multifaceted question that has not been fully resolved.[1,9,33,37,41]

The major disadvantage to colloid therapy is cost. Synthetic colloid preparations are expensive when compared to crystalloid solutions. Preparation of albumin or cruder colloid fractions (plasma) requires collection of blood and use of separation techniques, which may be unavailable. Although administration volume will be less when colloids are substituted or added to resuscitation protocols, cost will still exceed crystalloid solution resuscitation. Separation of outdated bank blood with collection of plasma components can diminish this cost. This technique is probably most economical at the present time.[23]

Colloids Available for Use

Colloids are both by-products of naturally occurring substances and specifically synthesized molecules. Natural colloid substances include plasma protein solutions and albumin. Synthetic preparations include dextrans and hydroxyethyl starch. Desirable properties of any colloid include freedom from pyrogens and antigens, stability for long-term storage, and maintenance of intravascular colloid osmotic pressure for several hours. Metabolism and excretion should not affect the animal and should not cause hemolysis or erythrocyte agglutination. Not all products fulfill all criteria; evaluation and production of synthetic materials has been developed in order to overcome objections noted with natural products. The major natural colloid substance in veterinary medicine is plasma protein. Plasma proteins may be commercially purchased or prepared from blood separation by centrifugation or gravitational methods. Plasma presses may be purchased and used with plastic bag blood containers (described below) to expedite fractionation. After separation, plasma is stored by freezing at $-4°C$ until required. Slow rewarming in a water bath at room temperature is preferred to rapid, high-temperature thawing. If anticipated use is within 24–48 hours after separation, then refrigeration storage is acceptable.[14,19]

Synthetic colloids are purchased from commercial sources. Dextrans and hydroxyethyl starch are two currently favored solutions. Both low- and high-molecular-weight dextrans are synthesized from microbiologic activity of *Leuconostic mesenteroides* B512 strain. Production of dextrans is controlled to produce low-molecular-weight (mean molecular weight 40,000 or Dextran 40) and high-molecular-weight (mean molecular weight 6–75,000 Dextran 60/75) varieties. Inclusion of polysaccharide chains is important in the production process in order to maintain preparation stability and aid in intravascular retention of dextrans. Hydroxyethyl starch is prepared by hydrolysis of corn or soybean substances. The hydrolyzed starch is attached to glucose units to provide satisfactory half-life within the intravascular space.[14]

BLOOD TRANSFUSION

Blood replacement can be essential to survival of trauma. No synthetic substitute has been shown to be satisfactory for replacement of fluid, colloid, and cellular deficits. Despite the potential lifesaving qualities of blood transfusion, inappropriate methods of collections, storage, and administration may minimize the benefit of transfusion and potentially increase the risk to the recipient. For these reasons, investigations in the past decade have centered on improved understanding of these aspects of blood therapy. Blood therapy must be considered in terms of immunologic compatibility, collection and storage technology, fractionation for specific component use, and adverse consequences of transfusion.

Compatibility

Blood is a living tissue. As with any tissue type, blood has the capability of evoking an immune response when transferred between individuals. The source of the immune response is twofold; cell surface antigens of the erythrocytes and plasma proteins plus antibody presence in the plasma fraction. Most domestic species have been evaluated and found to possess these antigen classes. Typing of blood has been performed in canine and feline species. Canine blood has been shown to possess one major cell surface antigen described as A type. Sixty percent of all dogs evaluated will possess this cell surface antigen. The cat has been shown to possess both A and B cell surface antigens with high frequency. It is important to note that canine A antigen is not the same as feline A antigen.[2,3,30]

The presence of erythrocyte antigens and the high incidence of plasma incompatibilities requires a typing procedure be performed prior to transfusion. Commercial laboratories can screen canine blood samples for detection of the presence of canine A antigen. Only dogs with documented absence of this antigen (A−) should be considered for donor use. Feline blood typing is currently being investigated. The practice of further cross-screening donor and recipient blood samples for compatibility (crossmatching) is unresolved. Crossmatching is practiced to determine presence of irregular antibodies other than major antigens. Studies of emergency transfusion of type-specific, uncrossmatched blood in man failed to demonstrate an increased incidence of transfusion reaction. While crossmatching should be performed on "elective" transfusion cases, many trauma animals receive type-specific blood replacement without crossmatching. It must be noted that corticosteroids may also be administered as a component of resuscitation, and their effect on inhibiting the incompatibility reaction is presently unknown. Partial crossmatching of recipient serum to donor erythrocytes may be quickly performed. Saline washed erythrocytes and recipient serum are added at room temperature, centrifuged, and evaluated for macroscopic agglutination. This procedure will screen most serum antibodies present in the recipient animal.[2,3,23,26,30]

Compatibility testing has significant effects on erythrocyte survival. Allogenic transfusion of compatible erythrocytes results in mean erythrocyte survival times approximating survival rates of autologous transfer. Transfusion of incompatible erythrocytes diminishes survival time to approximately one-third of autologous cell transfer. This survival period may produce equivocal benefit to the recipient as only 4- to 10-day survival times may be noted. Mean erythrocyte survival times were significantly lower with repeated transfusions in incompatible donor–recipient matches. Erythrocyte destruction occurred in less than seven days. This finding supports repeating transfusion procedures only with compatible donor cells. Prior unknown exposure to isoantibodies by previous transfusion episodes requires that screening procedures be performed during each transfusion episode.[6,22,27,35,43]

Collection and Storage of Blood

Collection techniques and procedures for blood collection vary with the situation. Under most circumstances, donor collection immediately prior to transfusion will occur. Conditions of high volume use may require practice of prior collection and remote storage. Each of these approaches can prove satisfactory if appropriate procedures and precautions are followed.

Donor animals should be regularly checked to prevent hematogenous transmission of infectious agents. In dogs, screening for *Dirofilaria immitis* is essential. In cats, screening for *Hemobartonella felis* and feline leukemia virus should occur. Routine vaccination schedules should be followed. Donor animals should ideally be segregated in a "closed" colony environment to minimize exposure to infectious agents. Good quality diets should be provided, as cyclical stress will occur from transfusion procedure. Periodic monitoring of packed cell volume and total plasma solids is minimal data base to evaluate post collection recovery. Animal size is important to consider. Medium to large size dogs of lean configuration provide better donors for collection procedures. Cats should be greater than 5 kg in weight. Neutering is recommended prior to use. Guidelines for donor collection should be established. Limiting collection to two units (1 L) of blood per 3-week period (20 percent blood volume) in dogs and 60 ml per 3 weeks in cats have proven workable in my experience. Exceeding these guidelines produces poor quality erythrocytes and potential donor aminal morbidity.[27]

The collection technique varies with the circumstance. Collection sites in the dog include external jugular and femoral veins and femoral artery. Collection sites in cats are the external jugular vein and cardiac puncture. Collection sites are clipped and prepared by scrubbing with surgical solutions. Animals may be manually restrained for the collection procedure or lightly anesthetized. For dogs, four to eight milligrams per pound thiamylyl sodium (Surital, Biotal) may be given. In cats, 3 to 5 mg per pound of ketamine HCl (Vetalar, Ketaset) may be administered. During collection, administration of volume replacement with crystalloid solutions is mandatory. In dogs, twice the collected volume is reinfused using balanced salt solutions. In cats, equivolume infusion is administered. Cardiovascular monitoring is provided during the collection procedure. All animals are monitored for a minimum of one hour post collection.

Vascular access is gained by introduction of a large bore (14–18 gauge) disposable needle into the lumen of the vessel. The needle is attached to the collection tubing and storage container. The operator should wear surgical gloves to minimize contamination during this procedure. After placement is confirmed, steady collection flow should be noted. Vacuum bottles provide pressure differential for collection. Polyethylene bags are gravity dependent for flow. I routinely place the collection bag 40–60 cm below the level of the animal. Slow gentle swirling or mixing should occur frequently during collection to prevent coagulation. Following collection, occlusion of the site by digital pressure is maintained for a minimum of 5 minutes to minimize hematoma formation. Small quantity collection in cats is performed in a similar fashion. A winged-needle tubing set (butterfly) of 18–19 gauge is usually selected. Syringe withdrawal using a 60 cc syringe is satisfactory in most cases. After collection, the blood is either used or immediately stored at 4°C until required. Maintenance of asepsis is essential at all stages of the collection. If loss of vascular access occurs or clotting is noted in the collection container, the blood is immediately discarded, and the procedure is restarted. The donor is monitored during recovery from anesthesia and checked 24 hours post collection, and weekly thereafter by collecting a PCV. This data is recorded on the blood container, along with donor identification. A chart is also recorded with the same information.

Storage

Collection of blood into an in vitro environment requires the presence of an anticoagulant medium to inhibit clotting and for inclusion of nutrient substrates favorable to continued erythrocyte metabolism. Several commercial preparations are available that fulfill these criteria. Alternate techniques of management may be used for short-term transfer storage. Limitations related to storage of blood exist with all currently available techniques. Newer methods of preservation show promise for improved survival times.

Commercially available solutions for storage medium include ACD (acid–citrate–dextrose), CPD (citrate–phophate–dextrose), CPD-A1 (citrate–phosphate–dextrose + adenine), and heparin. The anticoagulant component of all formulas except heparin is citrate. Citrate interacts with calcium ion to inhibit both intrinsic and extrinsic steps of the coagulation mechanism. Heparin acts by inhibiting factors VIII, IX, and XI of the coagulation profile. Heparin can be antagonized by thromboplastic substances liberated from blood during storage. Consequently, blood stored in heparin must be used within 48 hours after collection. Citrate effect is stable for long time periods; storage limitations are based on other factors[23,27,38] (Table 2-4).

Government regulations have been set regarding storage of blood. A requirement that at least seventy percent of the erythrocytes transfused remain in circulation for 24 hours after infusion has been described. Erythrocytes that survive for 24 hours posttransfusion will disappear at rates similar to other erythrocytes in matched donor–recipient transfusions. ACD solution has been shown to maintain this 70 percent confidence factor for 21 days postcollection. CPD solutions can extend this time to 28 days postcollection, although governmental regulations still stipulate a 21-day confidence.[23]

Several factors contribute to storage stability. Obligate metabolism of erythrocytes continues during storage, and substrate must be provided through inclusion of dextrose in the medium. Blood must be stored at 1°–6°C after collection to decrease the metabolic rate of erythrocytes. Storage at this temperature decreases the rate of glycolysis by 40 times, compared to room temperature. During storage, glucose is metabolized to lactate, and plasma pH falls. The presence of citric acid acts as a buffer that counteracts the decline in hydrogen concentration that occurs when blood is cooled. Low storage temperatures enhance exchange of sodium and potassium across the cell membrane, enhancing osmotic fragility. Progressive declines in erythrocyte concentration of high energy phosphate (ATP) and enzyme facilitating oxygen–hemoglobin interaction (2,3 diphosphoglycerate) contribute to limiting storage

Table 2-4. Storage Media Characteristics

Name	Composition	Medium pH	70% Erythrocyte Survival Time	Milliliters Solution to Preserve 100 ml Blood
Acid–Citrate–Dextrose (ACD)	1.47 g Dextrose 1.32 g Citrate salt 0.48 g Citric acid	5.0	28 days	6.6
Citrate–Phosphate–Dextrose (CPD)	1.61 g Dextrose 1.66 g Citrate salt 0.206 g Citric acid 0.14 g Monobasic sodium phosphate	5.5	28–35 days	7.15
Citrate–Phosphate–Dextrose–Adenine (CPD–Al)	CPD components plus 0.25–0.5 mM Adenine	5.5	35+ days	7.15
SMB	2.55 g Dextrose 2.63 g Sodium citrate 0.325 g Citric acid 0.222 g Sodium debasic phosphate 0.406 g Trisodium phosphate	7.0	49 days	17.5
Glycerol	35.0 g/dl Glycerol 2.88 g/dl Mannitol 0.065 g/dl Sodium chloride	7.0	Infinite	100

times for whole blood.[23,29] Newer formulations and techniques may improve blood storage capability. Addition of adenine to CPD solution (CPD-A1) improves erythrocytes survival by permitting ATP resynthesis. Higher glucose concentrations and adenine have improved storage capability to 35 days. Improved formulations of storage medium have increased canine erythrocyte survival to six weeks duration. Storing erythrocytes in glycerol–mannitol–sodium chloride medium has allowed long-term survival at a storage temperature of $-79°C$. These advances in whole blood preservation offer exciting alternatives in transfusion technology.[23,29,39,44]

Blood should be examined prior to administration for discoloration, hemolysis, and gross clotting. Questionable products should be discarded in order to avoid the risk of transfusion reaction.

Blood components may be separated from the collected blood unit. Red cell concentrates (60–80 percent erythrocytes) may be prepared by centrifugation or sedimentation of the blood over 24 hours. Plasma is then withdrawn by evacuated collection bottles (Travenol). Alternately, use of transfer packs allows direct separation by centrifugation and separation of gravitational drainage of sedimented erythrocytes. Viable platelets may be obtained by infusion of fresh blood or platelet-rich plasma. Platelets should be transfused within 12 hours after collection. Centrifugation of blood will allow platelet-rich plasma collection. Plasma and coagulation factors may be frozen up to one year at $-70°C$ after separation.[23,27]

Collection containers may factor in erythrocyte viability. Evacuated glass bottles draw blood quickly and require only gentle mixing of blood. However, blood drawn under negative pressure may be subjected to excessive shear stress, resulting in erythrocyte damage or hemolysis. Plastic bag collection is by passive gravitational flow; less erythrocyte injury occurs during the collection process. Containers are available in a 250 ml or 500 ml collection size with anticoagulant present. Plasma separation bottles are 100 ml in size. Ten ml of CPD solution can be mixed with 50 ml of feline blood for anticoagulation purposes.[23,27,39]

Indications for Blood Therapy

Blood transfusion is a substitution therapy that provides temporary support. However, the support from blood and blood products may be lifesaving. Therapeutic goals include restoration of oxygen carrying capacity, volume replacement, and administration of replacement coagulation factors. Whole blood is indicated when known blood loss, anemia, or coagulation defects exist. Anemia in the presence of normovolemia may best be treated by erythrocyte concentrates in order to minimize circulatory overexpansion. Plasma therapy is beneficial for restoration of circulating volume and coagulation factors, and improvement of plasma protein levels (colloid pressure). Fresh or frozen plasma may be used in coagulopathies, in hypoalbuminemic states, and in conjunction with intravascular volume resuscitation. Platelet-rich plasma is indicated in thrombocytopenia. Unfortunately, transfused platelets have short half life activity. Antiplatelet antibodies further diminish in vivo activity.[23,27]

Blood therapy is contraindicated in immune-mediated hemolytic disease unless life-threatening anemias exist. Incompatible donor–recipient match is a relative contraindication to transfusion. Interspecies transfusion is absolutely contraindicated.[27]

Administration of Blood

The severity and rapidity of blood loss will dictate transfusion management. The clinical cause of the anemia, the physical condition of the animal, and clinical judgment of the severity of blood loss are considered for replacement rates. Stored blood or components should be warmed to body temperature prior to administration. Warm water baths and periodic gentle mixing will aid in heat transfer. Water bath temperature should not exceed 46°C, as increased osmotic fragility of erythrocytes will occur at higher temperatures.[27,45]

Indwelling catheters should be used for blood administration. Aseptic preparation of venipuncture sites should be performed prior to catheter placement, and security of the catheter must be insured. Sites of catheterization have been previously described. An alternate administration route in puppies and kittens is intramedullary infusion following needle placement in the intertrochanteric fossa of the femur. A bone marrow needle with a removable stylet is preferred for this procedure.[27]

A filter must be used during administration of blood to remove aggregate debris. In our experience, a 40 micron in-line filter (Alpha Corp, Los Angeles, CA) has proven satisfactory. The design of the filter allows for adaptation to standard intravenous connectors. Constant monitoring during transfusion for nausea, vomiting, facial chemosis, coughing cutaneous erythema, and hypotension should be performed. Many of these signs may be masked by general anesthesia. We limit infusion rates to 20 ml/kg/hr with replacement of 20 percent of circulating volume per day unless acute blood loss demands rapid replacement. Syringe replacement in small size animals should not exceed 1 cc per minute. Administration may be accompanied by inclusion of an isotonic crystalloid solution to maintain venous patency during low flow rate blood infusion. The full effects of transfusion may not be realized for 12 to 24 hours.[27]

The volume of blood required for replacement can be determined from red cell mass. Knowledge of the donor packed cell volume and desired final hematocrit value is used in calculation. Normal blood volume in dogs is 85–90 mg/kg and 65–75 ml/kg in cats. An example is included in Table 2-5.[25,27]

Complications of Transfusion

Collection, handling, and storage of blood in vitro may pose potential problems with subsequent reinfusion. Problems associated with transfusion may be subdivided into in vitro changes, coagulation defects, physiologic response to

Table 2-5. Formula for Transfusion Volumes of Blood

Recipient weight = 30 kg
Recipient packed cell volume = 10%
Donor blood packed cell volume = 50%
Desired packed cell volume = 20%
1. Total blood volume of recipient
   90 ml/kg × 30 kg = 2700 ml
2. Existing erythrocyte mass
   2700 ml × 10% = 270 ml
3. Desired red cell mass
   2700 ml × 20% = 540 ml
4. Required red cell mass
   540 ml − 270 ml = 270 ml
5. Transfusion volume
   270 ml ÷ 50% = 540 ml

Adapted from Norsworthy GD: Blood transfusions in the cat. Feline Pract 7:29, 1977, and from O'Rourke LG: Practical blood transfusions. p. 408. In Kirk RW (ed) Current Veterinary Therapy. 8th Ed. WB Saunders, Philadelphia, 1983.

administration, and compatibility reactions. Each of these problems may be minimized or treated if prior knowledge of their occurrence is known.

In Vitro Changes. Storage media do not maintain ideal conditions. Changes in ATP concentration and activity of 2,3DPG occur. The change in 2,3DPG activity shifts the oxyhemoglobin dissociation curve to the left, theoretically inhibiting oxygen delivery to tissues under in vivo conditions. The magnitude of this change is related to volume and storage time. Experimental studies confirm the inhibition of oxygen delivery for as long as 9 hours after transfusion. Observation of increased cardiac output and cardiac work following transfusion in people has been noted. However, no specific evidence of tissue organ injury from hypoxia has been documented in any species.[24]

Progressive changes in blood pH occur during storage. Both ACD and CPD storage media have pH values in the acid range. Addition of blood to either medium changes blood pH to approximately 7.0–7.1. Erythrocyte metabolism further lowers pH by accumulation of lactic and pyruvic acids as end products of glycolysis. Blood pH declines to 6.6 by 21 days of storage. Part of this change is due to elevated PCO_2 levels of 150 to 220 mmHg. This is a result of a closed container without provision for escape of CO_2 accumulation. Even when restoration of normal PCO_2 values occur, acidosis is still present. However, buffering will occur in vivo and usually does not require supplemental bicarbonate administration. Metabolism of citrate from the anticoagulant may produce alkalosis. Therefore, empirical administration of bicarbonate with transfusion is not recommended unless coexisting metabolic acidosis is documented prior to transfusion.[24,29,39]

Coagulation Defects. Dilutional thrombocytopenia is the most frequent coagulation defect in man. At storage temperatures of 4°C, platelets are damaged sufficiently to be absorbed by the reticuloendothelial system soon after infusion. Remaining platelets have a reduced survival time. Platelet activity diminishes by 50 percent within 6 hours postcollection in cold blood. Activity

24 to 48 hours after storage begins is only 5 percent of normal. Multiple unit transfusion accentuates this observation, with hemorrhagic diathesis occurring if platelet levels fall below 50,000/mm³. Acutely induced thrombocytopenia appears to be less tolerated than chronically induced disease. Hemorrhagic tendencies must be monitored during multiple unit transfusions.[24]

Most coagulation factors remain stable during blood storage. Factors V and VIII have been shown in man to decrease to 15 to 50 percent of normal after 21 days of storage. The decrease per se has not been shown to cause clinically significant hemorrhagic diathesis, however, such deficiencies may be additive to other causes of bleeding.[24]

Disseminated intravascular coagulation (DIC) has been reported following shock and massive blood replacement. The pathogenesis of DIC differs little from other inciting causes. Release of tissue products, toxins, and thromboplastin may lead to generalized activation of the coagulation system. Hemolytic transfusion reaction may also be signaled by hemorrhagic diathesis.[24]

Diagnosis of coagulation defects is limited to laboratory evaluation. Thrombocytopenia, as previously noted, is the most frequent cause. Platelet count and administration of platelet-rich plasma can reverse the course of hemorrhage. Plasma fibrinogen levels may indicate the presence of DIC. Heparin therapy and other ancillary agents may be indicated as well as providing for consumed clotting factors (Factor VIII). Factor provision should be deferred until heparin therapy is given effective by reevaluating platelet numbers and fibrinogen levels. If a return toward normal values is noted along with decreased bleeding intensity, response to therapy is confirmed.[23,24]

Physiologic Responses. In addition to the development of in vitro acidemia during blood storage procedures, in vivo acidosis has been suggested. Massive blood transfusion (greater than five units in man) necessitates evaluation of arterial pH and PCO_2 levels. Correction should be performed only if severe metabolic acidosis is noted.[23,24]

Citrate intoxication has been documented during blood transfusion. Intravascular binding of ionized calcium is the mechanism involved. Rapid, multiple unit transfusion increases risk. Signs referable to citrate intoxication include hypotension, poor pulse quality, elevated central venous pressure, EKG abnormalities, and clotting deficiencies. These signs, if present, are transient; serum calcium levels return to normal as citrate is metabolized by the liver. Infusion rates of one unit of blood per 10-minute time period appears to increase risk. Slower infusion rates have a low incidence of citrate intoxication. If citrate intoxication is suspected, administration of calcium salts will minimize the clinical signs.[24]

Potassium levels also increase in stored blood and may be as high as 32 mEq/L in blood stored for 21 days. Elevation in serum potassium levels may be noted if administration rates exceed 120 ml/min. Extravascular diffusion and renal elimination account for potassium ion balance during transfusion.[23,24]

Infusion of cold (4°C) blood can decrease the recipient's body temperature. If core temperature decreases to less than 30°C, ventricular dysrhythmias and cardiac arrest can occur. Warming blood to body temperature prior to administration minimizes this risk. Immersion of the intravenous line in a warm water bath or attachment of a tubing length to a heating pad are two methods of adding heat. Warm baths to raise the blood temperature prior to administration is also effective.[10,24]

Controversy has surrounded the infusion of unfiltered debris in stored blood and the possibliity that it causes the development of respiratory distress. Platelet aggregates form during the second to fifth day of storage, with fibrin–leukocyte–platelet aggregates noted by day ten. If blood is used prior to this time, filtering during administration is probably unnecessary. The interaction between microaggregates and the development of respiratory distress after 10 days of storage is also debatable. Animal studies indicate that there is debris accumulation in the pulmonary microcirculation. It is hypothesized that release of vasoactive substances from the microaggregates may contribute to respiratory distress. However, clinical studies in man do not support this observation. Similar data has been determined in dogs. The question remains as to the value of in-line filters. We still require their use during transfusion to minimize infusion of macroaggregates (clots) which have been shown to be harmful to pulmonary function.[23,24]

Transfusion Reactions. The antibody to the A antigen in dogs and AB antigens in cats is a potent hemolysin. Transfusion of antigen to an unexposed recipient may result in: (1) no immediate reaction but future sensitivity, (2) a delayed response occurring 12 to 14 days posttransfusion, or (3) newborn hemolytic disease. Transfusion to a previously sensitized individual induces a rapid anamnestic hemolytic response. In addition, a transfusion reaction may be signified by urticaria, fever, hematuria, and anaphylaxis. Hemolysis may result from handling and administration or improper storage. Nephrotoxicity is a consequence of hemolytic by-products. Hypotension and hemorrhagic diathesis is noted in people. Therapy is directed at stopping the transfusion, instituting diuresis by mannitol and furosemide, alkalinizing urine to prevent formation of acid hematin, and monitoring for the development of DIC (Table 2.6).[24,27]

Sepsis. Improper handling of blood permits bacterial contamination and growth. Administration of contaminated blood may be accompanied by endotoxin production, resulting in endotoxic shock and DIC. Blood cultures should

---

Table 2-6. Treatment of Hemolytic Transfusion Reaction

1. Stop transfusion
2. Diuresis—75 to 100 ml/hr
   A. Administration of intravenous fluids
   B. 1–2 mg/kg Mannitol intravenously
   C. 0.5–1.0 mg/kg furosemide intravenously
3. Alkalinize urine. Administer sodium bicarbonate until urine pH is alkaline by analysis. Prevents acid hematin injury to renal tubules.
4. Determine platelet count, partial thromboplastin time, and serum fibrinogen level.
5. Prevent hypotension in order to insure adequate renal blood flow.

Adapted from Miller RD, Brzica SM. p. 908. In Miller RD (ed): Anesthesia. Churchill Livingstone, New York, 1981.

be performed if contamination is suspected after transfusion. Discard blood that may be contaminated prior to administration.[27]

AUTOTRANSFUSION

Autotransfusion is the technique of collection, processing, and reinfusion of the animal's own blood in order to maintain circulatory volume. Autotransfusion may be performed by several methods. Preoperative collection and storage can be performed on an elective, short-term basis, until the animal's surgical requirements arise. Immediate preoperative collection and hemodilution with crystalloid solution is another method described. Probably the most common form of autotransfusion in veterinary medicine is intraoperative blood salvage and retransfusion to decrease the necessity of homologous blood transfusion.[23]

Advantages

Autotransfusion may be performed under circumstances in which adequate quantities of stored homologous blood or typed donors are not available. Salvage of blood from body cavities or surgical sites minimizes the risk of transmitting infectious agents, prevents isoimmunization to cell, platelet, or protein antigens, minimizes graft-versus-host transfusion reactions, and provides a ready source of warm, fresh, compatible blood. Reinfusion of humoral agents may afford a greater immunologic response to the introduction of infectious agents than homologous blood transfusion.

The viability of erythrocytes is maintained better with autotransfusion. Experimental studies demonstrate similar survival times between erythocytes subjected to autotransfusion and normal erythrocytes. Levels of 2,3DPG have also been shown to be no different in autotransfused blood. Autotransfusion in many cases circumvents the complications related to administration of hypothermic blood. Finally, reinfusion of collected blood is valuable when the blood bank is inadequate and massive hemorrhage related to surgery is anticipated. Reinfusion of collected blood may prove lifesaving in those cases.[12,28]

Techniques of Autotransfusion

Under most circumstances, elective precollection for future use will not occur. Most indications for autotransfusion will be related to acute, closed cavity hemorrhage related to trauma or surgery. Autotransfusion is considered when sterile, uncontaminated wound hemorrhage is present, malignant cells are absent, and minimal contact of blood with the wound surface is anticipated. Several different techniques have been described for autotransfusion. Some systems and technology are not feasible for the average veterinary practice. The techniques described are adaptable to many practice settings.[12,28]

Autotransfusion requires a vacuum source for blood collection. In the simplest form, a large capacity sterile syringe is acceptable. A basic approach involves a collection catheter, intravenous tubing, a multiple port stopcock (four-way), and a blood filter. The syringe acts as an "aspirator" and infusion pump. A second syringe containing heparin is used to provide anticoagulant for collected blood. Details of the procedure are described in the listed reference.[12]

Most other techniques require the availability of an adjustable vacuum device. Electrical, water faucet, or central vacuum pumps can be a vacuum source. Several relatively inexpensive devices can be made or purchased. Five hundred ml glass bottles can be adapted for this purpose and are commercially available as chest drainage bottles. After sterilization, 37.5 ml of ACD solution or 2 percent sodium citrate is added. Attaching this bottle in series with the vacuum source and collection of blood by suction handle or implanted drain is performed. After collection, reinfusion occurs using in-line filtration of macroaggregates. Commercially available units (Sorenson Labs) use similar principles of collection and reinfusion. Their advantage is the use of plastic containers in place of glass. Cost is higher for the commercial apparatus. Other devices, used in people, incorporate suction devices and options for cell separation and washing. Their cost is prohibitive in veterinary medicine at the current time.[12,28]

Complications of Autotransfusion

Complications arise from the handling of blood during collection and reinfusion. In-line filtration of blood is recommended to prevent infusion of cell debris and microaggregates represented by fat, plasma lipoproteins, platelet and leukocyte clumps, and red cell–fibrin complexes. A dual filter technique of a 170 micron filter followed by a 40 micron filter has proven effective in this application. However, chemically active substances represented by serotonin, histamine, kinins, and catecholamines liberated from cell injury may interact to impair lung function in the posttransfusion period.[12]

Hemoglobinemia and hemoglobinuria may result from erythrolysis and hemoglobin liberation from mechanical injury. High negative pressure, foaming, and suction line turbulence are contributory. Therapy to prevent nephrotoxicity from free hemoglobin is described elsewhere.[12,28]

Alteration in coagulation may be noted posttransfusion. The potential for coagulation activation and development of DIC has been reported from autotransfusion. Thrombocytopenia, depression of factors V and VIII, and hypofibrinogenemia have been reported. However, the overall incidence is low.[12]

Sepsis and infusion of neoplastic cells have been documented with autotransfusion. Adherence to aseptic technique and knowledge of tumor presence minimizes risk.[12,28]

COMPLICATIONS OF INTRAVENOUS THERAPY

Specific contraindications and precautions have been described as a part of individual therapies. In addition, complications common to intravenous therapy have been documented. These factors are highlighted in the subsequent discussion.

Volume Overload

Acute overhydration may be encountered in aggressive fluid therapy protocols. Small weight animals may have a greater disposition toward overhydration because the margin of error in fluid administration is less than in larger animals. Studies in normal dogs and cats suggest that administration rates of 45 ml/lb/hr (90 ml/kg/hr) may be tolerated for brief time intervals (1 hour) without adverse reactions. Higher rates are tolerated in healthy dogs, as previously noted. Animals with significant cardiovascular disease, renal disease, Cushing's disease, pulmonary disease, or chronic depletion of fluid and electrolytes will be intolerant of high administration rates. The use of isotonic fluids such as 0.9 percent NaCl or lactated Ringer's solution may induce overhydration by retention of administered fluids within the intravascular space. Selection of fluid composition and administration rates should be made with a concern for these factors.[4,11]

Fluid administration rate must be monitored in high-risk patients. Measurement of central venous pressure will provide information regarding response to fluid administration rate. Central venous pressure (CVP) measurement has limitations in cases of isolated left heart failure or biventricular failure. Placement of a catheter into the pulmonary artery and monitoring of pulmonary capillary wedge pressure is valuable in these cases. The normal mean value for CVP is 0.5 cm H_2O, with values up to 10–15 cm H_2O noted in high administration rate volume replacement therapy. In general, it is best not to exceed CVP values of 10–12 cm H_2O except in emergency replacement protocols. Pulmonary capillary wedge pressures range from 2 to 20 mm Hg, and measurements can be used to estimate the tendency to form pulmonary edema by subcategorizing low (< 7 mm Hg), optimal (10–14 mm Hg), or elevated (>20 mm Hg) venous pressures and adjusting administration rates appropriately.[5]

Clinical signs of overhydration may include cough, moist rales on pulmonary field auscultation, tissue chemosis, hypothermia, and alteration in mental status (water intoxication). Reassessment of the goals of fluid therapy, calculated administration rate, and current patient status is imperative to prevent further complications. Therapy includes discontinuation of fluid administration, treatment for pulmonary edema (with oxygen, bronchodilators, diuretics), thermal support, and assessment of serum electrolyte values, if altered mentation is noted.[5,40]

Air Embolus

Venous air embolism is a dramatic complication of parenteral fluid administration. In people, infusion of 70 to 100 ml/sec to a total of over 200 ml is necessary to produce sudden death from cor pulmonale. Peripheral venous infusion using a nonpressurized system is unlikely to create conditions of large volume air introduction. However, smaller quantities may be introduced and can create complications under certain conditions. Use of flexible, nonventilated containers has been reported to minimize this complication, although administration set–catheter disconnection may allow air to enter. Central venous catheters pose a greater risk of air embolization. Aspiration of air during initial venipuncture can occur if the site of introduction is elevated relative to the level of the right atrium. Disconnection of the catheter hub–administration set interface may produce a similar complication.[21,42]

Particulate Matter

Particulate contamination occurs in commercially prepared solutions. The presence of rubber, metal fragments, fibers, mold, and plastics has been reported. The introduction of glass fragments from ampules opened to mix in the administered fluids, and coring of rubber injection ports from large-bore needles have also been described. Improved manufacturing techniques have diminished production-related contamination. Particles less than 50 microns in diameter are invisible to visual inspection. Particles as small as 12 microns may become entrapped in the pulmonary vascular bed.[21]

Little data regarding the implication of particulate matter infusion has been reported. Most likely, pulmonary entrapment of particles occurs in most cases. Reports have appeared regarding pulmonary hypertension and respiratory failure related to parenteral fluid administration. Particulate-mediated pulmonary edema in certain patients has been anecdotally suggested in the absence of other possible etiologies. The frequency of these findings has not been documented. This complication has been minimized by the use of in-line microfiltration.[21,42]

Chemical Contamination

Plasticizers used in the production of polyvinyl chloride containers have been reported to leach from the plastic into the solution and to accumulate in tissues. The significance of this finding, or long term implications of plasticizer toxicity have not been established.[21]

Admixture Incompatibility

Numerous studies of component incompatibility with added pharmacologic agents, electrolytes, acidifying or alkalinizing agents, and antimicrobials have been reported. Various charts and tables have been prepared by fluid manufacturers and others detailing admixture incompatibility. As a general rule, dextrose preparations are safe to add in most instances; electrolyte-containing solutions appear to be least compatible. The reader is referred to the references cited for further information on this topic.[21,42]

CHRONIC CATHETERIZATION AND INFUSION CARE

Administration of long-term intravenous therapy requires management and care of the implanted catheter. Depending upon the composition of the fluid to be infused and the goals of therapy, either peripheral or central implantation sites may be used. Irrespective of the site selected, the materials for catheter construction are the same for all commercial catheter designs, and knowledge of their biological reaction is useful in their selection and use.

Presently, materials available for catheter construction are derivatives of plastic monomers (polyethylene, polyvinyl) or fluorinated hydrocarbon derivatives (Teflon) and silicone (Silastic). All classes of material are flexible and biologically inert during chronic tissue implantation. However, numerous reports suggest that intravascular catheterization can be associated with complications, some of which may be related to the thrombogenic potential of these materials. Experimental data suggest that intraluminal introduction of any material evokes a rapid, platelet-mediated fibrin deposition on the external surface of the catheter. This may be noted as soon as 15 minutes after catheter placement and may "plateau' by 40 minutes. The fibrin sheath remains for the duration of catheter implantation and dislodges upon removal. The freed thrombi may migrate in the venous blood, resulting in subclinical pulmonary emboli. Heparin bonding to the catheter surface may briefly impede this fibrin aggregation; however, little advantage is realized with long-term implantation. Of the three materials, silicone has the lowest complication rate.[31,36]

Peripheral veins (cephalic, lateral tarsal) may be selected as cannulation sites when isotonic solutions are used. Hypertonic solutions using a dextrose base should be given at a central venous site. Percutaneous or surgical catheter implantation of the anterior vena cava via the external jugular vein is recommended.[8]

Placement techniques for long- and short-term cannulas differ. Wound care and implantation under aseptic conditions are critical to prevent complications. The proposed implantation site is prepared aseptically using three successive surgical scrubs of povidone-iodine with a water rinse after each scrub. After the final scrub, povidone-iodine solution or tincture of iodine should be applied. The site is barrier draped, and aseptic surgical technique is used for catheter placement. The operator wears gloves and performs catheter venipuncture using standard technique. An occlusive dressing with povidone-iodine ointment is placed over the venipuncture site, and the catheter is secured by either single ligature fixation to the skin using monofilament suture material or incorporation into a bandage dressing. A protective cover made of materials with minimal absorptive properties is applied, and continuous care is given. Every one or two days (or more frequently, if gross soiling is observed), the dressing is removed, and the venipuncture site is examined for erythema, induration, or other signs of infection. Using aseptic technique and surgical gloves, the skin around the wound is cleansed, and antibiotic or antimicrobial ointment and a new occlusive dressing is applied. Changing administration sets and venipuncture sites may be considered at this time.[13]

If wound care is appropriate and no clinical signs of catheter-related sepsis are noted, sequential venous rotation on a regular basis is not mandatory. Central venous placement of catheters in man has been maintained for as long as 55 days at one site with minimal complications when good catheter care was observed. Catheters have been implanted in dogs for as long as 100 days with appropriate care. Complications associated with chronic cannulation of peripheral veins have not been reported. If intimal injury from hypertonic solutions occurs, thrombophlebitis may be noted as soon as 48 to 72 hours after catheter placement.[15,47]

Continued nursing care is critical to maintenance of aseptic cannulation. The entire administration apparatus should be considered a "closed" system. Infusion catheters should not be used for the administration of pharmacological agents, blood sampling, and physiological measurements (eg, CVP). All connections and the administration set should be continuously disinfected. Each reservoir change should include cleaning of both the administration part of the bottle or bag and the coupling terminal of the administration apparatus with povidone-iodine. Each time a junction is disconnected, both ends should be cleansed prior to reattachment. The administration set and in-line filter should be changed every 24 hours or whenver it is contaminated. Any accidental disconnection should be treated as a septic break, and the administration apparatus and solution must be replaced. Contamination of the catheter site merits either replacement or rotation of the catheter to an alternate site. Although these procedures may seem extreme, sepsis in the debilitated patient has extreme consequences.[34]

CATHETER-RELATED COMPLICATIONS

Sepsis

Chronic catheter implantation has been reported to be associated with numerous complications, many of which are preventable with good catheter care. Catheter-related sepsis is the most frequent complication. Inadequate preparation or maintenance of the catheter site may result in bacterial or fungal sepsis. In the dog, gram-negative species account for the majority of contaminants in inadequately prepared venipuncture sites. Antibiotic ointments in the occlusive dressings inhibit bacterial growth but allow fungal multiplication. Occlusive dressings with antimicrobial agents (tame iodophor ointment) have been recommended to inhibit both bacterial and fungal sepsis.[7,20,34]

Unexplained pyrexia, leukocytosis, chills, glucose intolerance, alterations in level of consciousness, and generalized deterioration of the patient's condition are all clinical signs noted with sepsis. Hematogenous dissemination from a septic anatomical site may be an additional factor. It should be determined whether sepsis is catheter-related or whether it arises from a secondary anatomical site. Catheter-related sepsis is usually noted shortly after implantation. Fibrin sheaths surround the catheter during the first 3 to 5 days following implantation. After this time, bacterial colonization of the catheter from remote sites is difficult. Introduction of cutaneous organisms during venipuncture and migration from the venipuncture site down the catheter shaft have been suggested. Removal of the administration system and solution container is mandatory. Antibiotic infusion through a contaminated catheter is not therapeutic. After removal, culture of the catheter, administration apparatus, and solution is suggested. In man, removal of a contaminated catheter is accompanied by remission of pyrexia in 12 to 24 hours. A new catheter is aseptically implanted at an alternate site. In cases of a refractive pyrexia (greater than 24 hours) or secondary catheter sepsis from a remote anatomical site, antibiotics should be administered, if not previously initiated for other reasons. Blood cultures should also be considered in cases of refractive fever.[7,20,34]

Thrombophlebitis

Thrombophlebitis and vascular occlusion have been associated with chronic catheterization. Chemical and mechanical factors may predispose the patient to this complication. Hypertonic solutions may induce endothelial irritation and stimulate platelet accumulation. Peripheral veins are especially susceptible, owing the disparity between the catheter diameter and the venous lumen. This disparity results in low blood flow and retarded dilution of hypertonic solutions, causing vascular irritation and thrombophlebitis. Mechanical injury to the endothelium from catheter placement may be interactive.[34,35,47,48]

Several recommendations have been proposed in order to minimize thrombophlebitis. A study comparing four catheter materials showed a lower incidence of complications when fluoroethylenepropylene or Silastic was used as a catheter material. These materials are superior to plastic, polyvinylchloride, and tetrafluoroethylene as a catheter material. The addition of heparin (500 units) and hydrocortisone (1 mg/L of parenteral solution) decreased thrombophlebitis in peripheral veins. In-line filtering to prevent infusion of particulate matter was reported to decrease vascular complications. Venipuncture may also create mechanical injury and tissue thromboplastin release. This injury secondarily creates platelet aggregation and promotes thrombus formation.[44]

REFERENCES

1. Appel PL, Shoemaker WC: Evaluation of fluid therapy in adult respiratory failure. Crit Care Med 9:862, 1981
2. Auer L, Bell K: The AB blood group system of cats. Anim Blood Grps Biochem Genet 12:287, 1981

3. Auer L, Bell K, Coates S: Blood transfusion reactions in the cat. J Am Vet Med Assoc 180:729, 1982

4. Bjorling DE, Rawlings CA: Relationship of intravenous administration of Ringer's lactate solution to pulmonary edema in halothane-anesthetized cats. Am J Vet Res 44:1000, 1983

5. Bonagura JD: Fluid and electrolyte management in the cardiac patient. Vet Clin North Am 12:501, 1982

6. Brown IW, Eadie GS: An analytical study of in vivo survival of limited population of animal erythrocytes tagged with radioiron. J Gen Physiol 36:327, 1952

7. Burrows CF: Inadequate skin preparation as a cause of intravenous catheter-related infection in the dog. J Am Vet Assoc 180:747, 1982

8. Carter JM, Freedman AB: Total intravenous feeding in the dog. Am J Vet Res 171:71, 1977

9. Civetta JM: Intravenous fluid therapy: colloid vs. crystalloid. Refresher Courses, Am Soc Anesth 209, 1978

10. Copping JW, Mather GS, Winkler JM: Physiological responses to the administration of cold, room temperature, and warm balanced salt solutions in hemorrhagic shock in dogs. Surgery 71:206, 1972

11. Cornelius LM, Finco DR, Culver DH: Physiologic effects of rapid infusion of Ringer's lactate solution into dog. Am J Vet Res 39:1185, 1978

12. Crowe DT: Autotransfusion in the trauma patient. Vet Clin North Am 10:581, 1980

13. Deutsch S: Effects of anesthetics on the kidney. Surg Clin North Am 55:775, 1975

14. Doenicke A, Grote B, Lorenz W: Blood and blood substitutes. Br J Anaesth 49:681, 1977

15. Dudrick SJ, Wilmore DW, Vars HM: Long-term parenteral nutrition with growth in puppies and positive nitrogen balance in patients. Surg Forum 18:356, 1967

16. Furman EB: Intraoperative fluid therapy. In Furman EB (ed): The Anesthesiologist's Role in Pediatric Acute Care. Int Anesthesiol Clin 13:133, 1976

17. Gieseke AH: Perioperative fluid therapy—crystalloids. p 865. In Miller RD (ed): Anesthesia. Churchill Livingstone, New York, 1981

18. Goldberger E: A Primer of Water, Electrolyte, and Acid–Base Syndromes, 5th Ed. Lea and Febiger, Philadelphia, 1975

19. Jennings PB, Whitten NJ, Sleeman HK: The Diagnosis and Treatment of Shock in the Critical Care Patient. p. 486. In Sattler FP, Knowles RP, Whittick WG (eds): Veterinary Critical Care. Lea and Febiger, Philadelphia, 1981

20. Kaminski MV, Harms DF: Prolonged uncomplicated intravascular catheterization. Am J IV Ther 3:19, 1976

21. Lawson DH, Henry DA: Intravenous fluid therapy. J Maine Med Assoc 68:432, 1977

22. Marion RS, Smith JE: Survival of erythrocyte after autologous and allogenic transfusion in cats. J Am Vet Med Assoc 183:1437, 1983

23. Miller RD, Brzica SM: Blood, blood component, colloid and autotransfusion therapy. In Miller RD, (ed): Anesthesia. Churchill Livingstone, New York, 1981

24. Miller FD: Problems posed by transfusion. In Orkin FK, Cooperman LE (eds): Complications in Anesthesiology. JB Lippincott, Philadelphia, 1983

25. Norsworthy GD: Blood transfusion in the cat. Feline Pract 7:29, 1977

26. Orlin JB: Emergency blood transfusion: assessing the risks. Crit Care Monitor 3: 12, 1983

27. O'Rourke LG: Practical Blood Transfusions. p 408. In Kirk RW (ed): Current Veterinary Therapy. 8th Ed. WB Saunders Co., Philadelphia, 1983

28. Orr MD: Autotransfusion: Intraoperative therapy. In Stehling LC (ed): Techniques of Blood Transfusion. Int Anesthesiol Clin 20:97, 1982
29. Ou D, Mahaffey E, Smith JE: Effect of storage on oxygen dissociation of canine blood. J Am Vet Med Assoc 167:56, 1975
30. Perman V, Schall WD: Diseases of the red blood cells. p. 1983. In Ettinger S (ed): Textbook of Veterinary Internal Medicine. 2nd Ed. WB Saunders, Philadelphia, 1983
31. Peters WR, Bush WH, McIntyre RD: The development of fibrin sheath in indwelling venous catheters. Surg Gynecol Obstet 137:43, 1973
32. Puri VK, Paidpaty B, White L: Hydroxyethyl starch for resuscitation of patients with hypovolemia and shock. Crit Care Med 9:833, 1981
33. Rodman GH, Kirby RR: Post-traumatic respiratory failure: role of fluid therapy. p. 119. In Brown BR (ed): Contemporary Anesthesia Practice. Vol. 6. FA Davis, Philadelphia, 1983
34. Ryan JA, Abel RM, Abbott DM et al: Catheter complications in total parenteral nutrition. N Engl J Med 290:757, 1974
35. Schalm OW, Jain NC, Carroll EJ: Veterinary Hematology. 3rd Ed. Lea and Febiger, Philadelphia, 1975
36. Schlossman D: Thrombogenic properties of vascular catheter material in vivo. Acta Radiol 14:186, 1973
37. Shoemaker WC: Crystalloids, colloids, and blood products. Refresher Courses, Am Soc Anesth 126B, 1981
38. Smith HA, Jones TC, Hunt RD: Veterinary Pathology. 4th Ed. Lea and Febiger, Philadelphia, 1972
39. Smith JE, Mahaffey E., Board P: A new storage medium for canine blood. J Am Vet Med Assoc 172:701, 1978
40. Stamp GL: Metabolic response to trauma. In Zaslow IM (ed): Veterinary Trauma and Critical Care. Lea and Febiger, Philadelphia, 1984
41. Staub NC: Pathophysiology of microembolism lung injury. Refresher Courses, Am Soc Anesth 302, 1983
42. Stephen M, Loewenthal J, Wong J: Complications of intravenous therapy. Med J Aust 2:557, 1976
43. Swisher SN, Young LE, Trabold N: In vitro and in vivo studies of the behavior of canine erythrocyte isoantibody systems. Ann NY Acad Sci 97:15, 1962
44. Turco SJ: Infusion phlebitis: pathogenesis remains unclear, but preventive measures emerge from many studies. Crit Care Monitor 2:6, 1982
45. Valeri CR, Valeri DA, Gray A et al: Horse red blood cells frozen with 20% glycerol and stored at −150°C for five years. Am J Vet Res 44:2200, 1983
46. Van der Walt JH, Russell WJ: Effect of heating on the osmotic fragility of stored blood. Br J Anaesth 50:815, 1978
47. Virgilio RW, Smith DE Zarins CK: Balanced electrolyte solutions: experimental and clinical studies. Crit Care Med 7:98, 1979
48. Wilmore DW, Dudrick SJ: Safe long-term venous catheterization. Arch Surg 98:256, 1969

3 | Anesthesia for the Emergency Surgical Patient

John A. E. Hubbell

PREANESTHETIC CONSIDERATIONS

A thorough preoperative examination is essential for safe anesthetic management of the emergency surgical patient.

Signalment

The signalment gives clues to the anesthetic requirement of the patient. Anesthesia in cats is associated with greater mortality than anesthesia in the dog.[1] Cats and small breed dogs (less than 20 pounds) tend to lose more heat during anesthesia, thus hypothermia may be an operative and postoperative concern. Older dogs are more likely to have renal and hepatic compromise and may be difficult to maintain with inhalation anesthesia due to decreases in respiratory function.[12] Brachycephalic breeds such as the English bulldog may benefit from anticholinergic drug administration to decrease salivary secretion, helping to maintain a clear airway. Sight hounds, such as the greyhound and Borzoi, have a decreased percentage of body weight as fat and may have a prolonged recovery following thiobarbiturate administration.

History

The history provides important information relative to the physiological state of the animal. A dog with a history of acute vomiting may have metabolic alkalosis due to the loss of gastric acid. Chronic vomiting is more often associated with hypokalemia, hypochloremia, and metabolic acidosis. Increased water consumption and increased frequency of urination may be indicative of renal disease diabetes mellitus, or other endocrine diseases.

Food consumption within 8 hours of presentation is an indication for postponing surgery, if possible. The incidence of emesis or regurgitation is greatly increased by the presence of food material in the stomach. Ingesta present in the airway may cause acute respiratory obstruction or pneumonia postoperatively. Anesthesia in the presence of a full stomach requires rapid induction, endotracheal intubation, and assisted ventilation with a cuffed endotracheal tube. A cuffed endotracheal tube will assure a patent airway and minimize aspiration of foreign material. An alternative approach is to administer drugs (apomorphine, morphine, xylazine) that cause emesis, partially emptying the stomach.

The animal's mental state may give evidence of metabolic disease or cranial trauma. The comatose patient is a poor candidate for anesthesia and requires dramatically decreased doses of anesthetic drugs. Determination of the cause of coma prior to anesthesia is essential. Phenothiazine tranquilizers should be avoided in a seizing patient or one with a history of seizures, because the drugs lower the seizure threshold.

Physical Exam

A thorough physical exam emphasizing the cardiovascular, respiratory, and central nervous systems is required prior to the induction of anesthesia.

Cardiovascular System. The cardiovascular physical exam consists of auscultation of the chest, palpation of the peripheral pulse, examination of the color of mucous membranes, and determination of the capillary refill time. Cardiac rhythm and rate should be determined. Animals with pain or in shock may have increased heart rates, while hyperkalemia or cranial trauma may cause bradycardia. Cardiac rhythm disturbances, primarily ventricular extrasystoles, may occur in the patient with chest trauma, central nervous system disease, or gastric torsion. Variable intensity cardiac sounds, tachycardia, bradycardia, or irregularity of cardiac sounds may indicate the presence of cardiac dysrhythmias, thus, further investigation is required prior to induction of anesthesia.

Palpation of the pulse strength and regularity indicate the mechanical function of the myocardium, the fluid status of the patient, and the tone of the peripheral vasculature. The color of mucous membranes is an indicator of the oxygenation of the patient. Hypoxemia in patients with normal hemoglobin levels is manifested by cyanosis. Anemic animals can be hypoxic but not cyanotic, due to decreased hemoglobin levels. Blood loss can cause the mucous membranes to become pale, while toxemia or hypercarbia causes an injected or "brick red" appearance. Capillary refill time is an indicator of tissue perfusion. Hypoperfusion causes increases in capillary refill time beyond the normal 1.5 to 2 seconds.

Respiratory System. The respiratory system is evaluated by measuring the respiratory rate and by percussing and auscultating chest. Increased respiratory rate may indicate pulmonary insufficiency or may simply occur due to excitement. Slow respiratory rates or altered respiratory patterns may result from cranial trauma due to increased intracranial pressure or drug overdose. Absent or diminished respiratory sounds on auscultation may indicate consolidation of lung lobes, or displacement of the lungs away from the chest wall. Displacement of the lungs from the chest wall can be caused by air or fluid within the chest or the presence of a diaphragmatic hernia. Abnormal lung sounds include increased bronchovesicular sounds, wheezes, and crackles. Increased lung sounds may be the result of pneumonia or pulmonary edema. Increased lung sounds are often overinterpreted in young or thin patients, due to the lack of body fat. The presence of intestinal sounds in the thorax may indicate the presence of a diaphragmatic hernia, although this is inconsistent and must not be the sole criterion used to diagnose this problem.

Percussion is an additional way of assessing the respiratory system. Hyperresonancy is generally the result of a pneumothorax. A dull, hyporesonant percussion sound is an indication of an abnormal fluid density in the chest. Causes of hyporesonant percussion sounds include hemothorax, pyothroax, chylothorax, and diaphragmatic hernia. Alterations from the normal lung sounds or changes in percussion sounds may indicate thoracic lesions and should be investigated further.

The surface of the thorax should be examined for lacerations or wounds that penetrate the chest cavity. Pain elicited on palpation of the chest may indicate fractured ribs. A "free floating" portion of the chest wall showing paradoxical movement (flail chest) indicates severe chest wall trauma. Pulmonary edema and contusions generally accompany this condition and must be evaluated carefully prior to any anesthetic episode.

Neurologic System. The central nervous system (CNS) should be evaluated for evidence of cranial trauma. Cranial trauma often causes an alteration in the level of consciousness and increases in cerebrospinal fluid pressure. Physical signs of increased cerebrospinal fluid pressure include ocular papilledema, bradycardia, and altered respiration. Seizure activity may indicate cranial trauma, hypoxia, or toxin ingestion.

Musculoskeletal System. Palpation of large fracture hematomas upon examination of the musculoskeletal system may indicate significant blood loss. Trauma to the front limbs indicates probable trauma to the chest. Trauma to any part of the body in small dogs and cats possibly indicates trauma to the chest. Fractures of the mandible or maxilla may cause respiratory dyspnea and can make intubation difficult. A tracheotomy may be necessary to allow intubation. Cervical dislocations or fractures must be handled carefully so that there is no displacement during intubation or when the animal is relaxed under anesthesia.

Urinary System. Animals with pelvic trauma should be evaluated for the presence of a ruptured bladder. Rupture of the urinary tract can cause distension of the abdomen and electrolyte abnormalities, primarily hyperkalemia and hyponatremia. Uremia may accentuate the effects of some anesthetic agents (barbiturates, diazepam) due to its effect of decreasing protein binding. It also causes various degrees of CNS depression. The amount of anesthetic agent used must be decreased accordingly, if uremia is present. Palpation of a small but intact bladder may indicate dehydration.

Digestive System. The digestive system should be evaluated for distension of the abdomen, the presence or absence of feces, the presence of blood in the feces, and for signs of vomiting. Distension of the abdomen can cause respiratory embarrassment due to increased intra-abdominal pressures. Gas distension of the abomen should be relieved prior to induction of anesthesia.

Clinical Pathology

Abnormalities discovered during the physical examination indicate the need for further preoperative workup of the patient. A packed cell volume (PCV) and total protein (TP) are simple tests that reveal much about the fluid status of the patient. Packed cell volume is used as an index of the oxygen-carrying capacity of the blood and the hydration of the patient. Total plasma protein is an indicator of plasma oncotic pressure, an important factor in the maintenance of intravascular fluid volume. Packed cell volume and TP are increased during dehydration. Accurate estimation of blood loss is difficult in animals, because packed cell volume and total protein may not change acutely following hemorrhage. If the preinjury weight of the animal is known, the animal can be weighed when presented and the difference determined. The difference between preinjury and postinjury weight represents the weight of blood lost. Unfortunately, this is rarely possible. Adequacy of fluid replacement is best assessed by evaluating the patient's response to therapy. Following blood loss, fluids should be given until the animal's pulse strengthens and the heart rate decreases to near normal. The maximum amount of fluid to be replaced acutely is one blood volume (90 ml/kg). Administration of polyionic solutions will cause a fall in PCV and TP. Total plasma protein should not be allowed to fall below 3.5 g/dl, because plasma proteins, in particular albumin, are, in part, responsible for retaining fluid within the vascular space. The plasma proteins cannot hold additional fluid within the vascular volume, and edema occurs if TP is diluted below 3.5 g/dl. Further fluid volume replacement must be done using plasma or whole blood if TP falls to 3.5 g/dl.

The preoperative hemogram in emergency patients frequently demonstrates a mild leukocytosis, neutrophilia, and a lymphopenia that can be attributed to the effects of excitement and stress. Elevations of the white blood cell count (WBC) above 13,000 cells/μl or decreases below 5,500 cells/μl require further evaluation.

Serum electrolyte concentrations should be measured in patients with abnormal physical examinations that suggest metabolic disease. Animals with ruptured gastrointestinal tracts or urinary tracts can have severe electrolyte abnormalities, including hyperkalemia, hyponatremia, and hypochloremia. Animals with diarrhea lose bicarbonate and body fluids, thus they can become metabolically acidotic. Metabolic acidosis causes potassium to shift out of the cells, which may result in hyperkalemia. Hyperkalemia is potentially the most devastating electrolyte abnormality in the anesthesia patient. Hyperkalemia causes muscle weakness, cardiac atrioventricular conduction disturbances, and decreases in heart rate. The electrocardiogram in hyperkalemia includes peaked, narrow T waves, shortened Q–T intervals, loss of the P wave, and widening of the QRS complex. Hyponatremia can potentiate the cardiac effects of hyperkalemia by decreasing the velocity of cardiac depolarization. Hyperkalemia can occur during acidosis; following muscle trauma, renal disease, Addison's disease; or as the result of drug administration.

Serum calcium concentrations are of concern especially in the bitch presented for Caesarian section. Hypocalcemia can occur prior to delivery or following delivery, as milk production increases. Symptoms of hypocalcemia include rapid breathing, nervousness, restlessness, excessive salivation, clonic and tonic spasms, and convulsions. Treatment should include control of the seizures and controlled infusion of calcium solutions.

Serum chemistries should be performed if the prior workup indicates organic disease. Animals, particularly the neonate, that are weak or comatose should be evaluated for hypoglycemia. Older dogs should have their kidney function checked by measuring serum creatinine or blood urea nitrogen levels. Urinalysis may be helpful in determining the concentrating ability of the kidney and the presence or absence of glomerular disease. Liver enzymes may often be elevated in surgical emergencies, especially in those involving trauma. Elevation in liver enzymes is not a good indicator of liver disease.[4] Dye clearance tests such as bromsulphalein clearance are better tests for the active capacity of the liver.

Blood pH and blood gases measure the acid–base balance. Traumatized animals often suffer a period of shock and hypoperfusion of the tissues. With the hypoperfusion of tissues, lactic acid may build up due to anaerobic metabolism. Blood pH and blood gases are the only true determinants of the animal's acid–base balance. A device for measuring the total carbon dioxide in the blood can be used in practice as an index of serum bicarbonate. The total carbon dioxide analyser is used to assess the metabolic component of acid–base derangements. Arterial pH and blood gases must be measured, if an assessment of ventilatory adequacy is required. Patients with respiratory depression, pneumonia, or trauma to the thorax may have respiratory embarrassment and thus are candidates for arterial blood gas analysis.

Further Preanesthetic Diagnostics

One-third of small animals sustaining trauma to the front or rear legs may have thoracic injuries that include pulmonary contusions, diaphragmatic hernia, rib fractures, and pneumothorax.[14] Animals admitted following trauma, with any evidence of pulmonary dysfunction on physical examination, should have thoracic radiographs taken and evaluated prior to anesthesia. If thoracic radiographs are not available, the animal should be assumed to have chest trauma and a pneumothorax. Abdominal radiographs may be helpful in some animals with abdominal trauma, especially where a ruptured bladder or retroperitoneal hemorrhage is suspected.

A significant number of small animal trauma patients have cardiac arrhythmias including premature ventricular contractions and ventricular tachycardia.[7] A preoperative electrocardiogram should be performed on patients having irregular heart rates, pulse deficits, or abnormal cardiac sounds on the cardiovascular physical examination. Animals with frequent premature ventricular contractions or ventricular tachycardia should not be anesthetized until the arrhythmias have been converted and the animal has been stabilized in normal sinus rhythm.

ANESTHETIC CONSIDERATIONS

The Patient with General Trauma

The metabolic response to trauma has been discussed elsewhere in this volume. In general, the traumatized patient has some degree of circulatory shock. An increased heart rate, weak peripheral pulses, and rapid shallow respirations are signs of a hypovolemic, shocky patient. Hypovolemia leads to centralization of the blood volume, decreased perfusion of peripheral tissues, and metabolic acidosis.

It is imperative to stabilize the patient prior to the induction of anesthesia. Polyionic solutions or blood should be administered in order to restore blood volume. If hypotension persists following fluid replacement, drugs to increase cardiac output may be required. Dopamine (Inotropin) (1–5 μg/kg/min) and dobutamine (Dobutrex) (1–5 μg/kg/min) promote perfusion by increasing the force of myocardial contraction. These agents should not be used in the absence of adequate fluid replacement. Response to therapy can be further assessed by measuring urinary output. Urinary output is a good indicator of organ perfusion and should be approximately 1–2 ml/kg/hour.

Drugs selected for use in the patient with general trauma should provide anesthesia with minimal cardiovascular depression. It must be realized that there are no safe anesthetics or safe anesthetic techniques, there are only safe anesthetists.

Anesthetic Drugs to Avoid

Animals that have sustained trauma are usually depressed, hence they seldom require heavy sedation prior to anesthesia. Tranquilizers in general should be avoided in trauma patients. Xylazine (Rompun) and phenothiazine derivatives produce more sedation than is required in trauma patients and should not be used in patients with cardiovascular compromise. The sympathetic nervous system mediates increases in cardiac output and arteriolar constriction as a normal response to hypovolemia and hypotension. Phenothiazine tranquilizers induce alpha adrenergic blockade and may augment hypotension, thus hypovolemic animals may be especially sensitive to phenothiazine administration. Xylazine decreases heart rate, thus normal reflex-induced increases in heart rate and cardiac output are blunted.

Useful Anesthetic Drugs

Adequate preoperative sedation in most trauma patients can be produced using IV diazepam (Valium 0.2 mg/kg). Diazepam produces calming with minimal cardiopulmonary depression. Diazepam potentiates the action of analgesics but provides no analgesia itself. Diazepam prevents seizures, thus it is especially useful in the patient suffering cranial trauma.

Narcotics provide analgesia and mild sedation with minimal cardiovascular depression. Narcotics can be used to supplement inhalation anesthesia or combined with tranquilizers to provide balanced anesthesia. Morphine, oxymorphone (Numorphan), and fentanyl (Sublimase) are potent narcotics that can be used subcutaneously (SC), intramuscularly (IM), or intravenously (IV) in the dog. Narcotics, although rarely used in the cat, can be employed at low doses. Narcotics are respiratory depressants, thus ventilation should be monitored. Neuroleptanalgesic combinations such as fentanyl citrate–droperidol (Innovar–Vet) can be used to provide tranquilization with analgesia.

Ultrashort-acting barbiturates such as thiamylal or thiopental can be used safely in patients with cardiovascular compromise if doses are strictly limited to the amount of drug required to induce anesthesia. Larger doses of barbiturates as the sole anesthetic agent are discouraged because of the profound cardiopulmonary depression that can be produced. A newer technique for the induction of anesthesia includes the use of thiobarbiturates followed by an IV bolus of lidocaine hydrochloride.[11] The combination of thiobarbiturates and lidocaine produces anesthesia with reduced cardiopulmonary depression due to the reduction in thiobarbiturate dose.

Etomidate (Amidate), a rapidly acting nonbarbiturate hypnotic is useful for the induction of general anesthesia in the trauma patient. Etomidate produces hypnosis with minimal cardiopulmonary depression. Etomidate is presently available only for use in people but has been shown to be very safe and efficacious in the dog.[8] Etomidate is prohibitively expensive for routine clinical use at this time.

Inhalation anesthetics can provide complete anesthesia for the patient. Inhalation anesthetics produce dose-dependent cardiopulmonary depression. Nitrous oxide can be used to supplement the analgesia of the other more potent agents, if there is no thoracic compromise. Inhalation anesthetics are delivered in oxygen, which is of benefit to the patient with cardiopulmonary compromise. Severely compromised patients may not tolerate anesthetic levels of the inhalation anesthetics. In severely compromised patients, narcotics can be used to supplement inhalation agents and allow a reduction in inhalation anesthetic level. Fentanyl can be administered IV at doses of 0.002–0.005 mg/kg, repeated at 15- to 20-minute intervals as required. The choice of inhalant anesthetic depends upon the patient, the clinican's familiarity with the drugs, and the cost of the anesthetic.

Isoflurane (Forane) is the best inhalation anesthetic available. It produces the least cardiovascular depression of all the potent inhalation agents. Isoflurane and enflurane (Ethrane), another new inhalation agent, produce rapid induction and recovery due to their low blood–gas solubility. Isoflurane and enflurane do not potentiate catecholamine-induced cardiac arrhythmias. Enflurane is a more potent respiratory depressant than isoflurane; thus, ventilation should be supported. Unfortunately, at this time enflurane and isoflurane are 10 to 14 times as expensive as halothane and methoxyflurane (Metofane); thus, they are impractical for general use.

Halothane and methoxyflurane, while not ideal, are very useful anesthetic agents. Both agents have advantages and disadvantages. Either agent may be too potent a cardiopulmonary depressant at anesthetic concentrations in patients suffering general trauma. Inhalation anesthetic concentrations should be reduced and IV narcotics used to supplement analgesia if the patient does not tolerate anesthetic levels of inhalation anesthetic agents.

SPECIAL PROBLEMS IN ANESTHESIA

The Patient with Head Trauma

The patient with head trauma should be thoroughly evaluated prior to anesthesia. Patients with altered respiration, bradycardia, and ocular papilledema may have increased intracranial pressure. Pupillary size and light reflexes should be examined. The patient with increased intracranial pressure is a poor candidate for anesthesia. Mannitol (0.5–2 g/kg) should be used to reduce intracranial pressure due to edema. Diuretics (Lasix) and corticosteroids can also be used to reduce edema and stabilize cell membranes. Following reduction of intracranial pressure and stabilization of the patient, anesthesia may be induced.

Inhalation anesthetics, in general, should be avoided in the patient with head trauma. Inhalation anesthetics increase brain blood flow, thus increasing intracranial pressure.[15] Inhalation agents can only be used if the patient is hyperventilated prior to the inhalation agent being introduced. Hyperventilation causes cerebrovascular vasoconstriction, reducing brain blood flow and thus intracranial pressure. Patients with head trauma should be hyperventilated whether or not inhalation anesthetics are used. Nitrous oxide can be used to supplement other anesthetic techniques.

Patients with head trauma are often depressed and do not usually require heavy sedation. Diazepam (IV, 0.2 mg/kg) is a good choice in these patients, because it provides light sedation with minimal cardiopulmonary depression. Diazepam is also useful in controlling seizures that may occur after head trauma.

Barbiturates are a good choice to induce anesthesia in the patient with head trauma. Controversy exists relative to the barbiturates' protective effects on the brain following cerebral injury.[13] Barbiturates lower cerebral metabolic rate and thus may decrease the oxygen demand of brain tissue. Ultrashort-acting barbiturates (thiopental, thiamylal) are used to induce the patient to general anesthesia. Pentobarbital can be used to provide sedation and hypnosis. Respiration should be supported following barbiturate administration because hypoventilation can lead to hypercarbia and increases in intracranial pressures due to cerebrovascular vasodilation.

Narcotics are used to good advantage in the patient with head trauma. The narcotics provide some sedation and analgesia. Narcotics are respiratory depressants, so respiration should be supported. At the end of surgery, narcotics may have to be reversed with narcotic antagonists such as naloxone (Narcan).

The Patient with Chest Trauma

The patient with chest trauma may or may not have external evidence of trauma. The lesions of chest trauma may include myocarditis, pneumothorax, tension pneumothorax, hemothorax, fractured ribs, lacerated lungs, and diaphragmatic hernia, alone or in combination. Any animal suffering trauma should be evaluated for thoracic compromise. If there is any evidence of thoracic compromise on physical exam, a thoracic radiograph should be taken and evaluated. Animals with irregular heart rates or pulse deficits should be evaluated for cardiac arrhythmias.

Pneumothorax causes respiratory embarrassment due to the inability of the patient to expand the lungs. Tension pneumothorax can cause cardiac dysfunction as well as respiratory embarrassment due to decreases in venous return resulting from increases in intrathoracic pressure. Decreases in venous return result in decreases in cardiac output. Animals with pneumothorax or tension pneumothorax should have a chest tube placed prior to the induction of anesthesia in order to relieve pressure in the chest and expand the lungs. Respiration should be supported in patients with respiratory dysfunction. Care must be taken when ventilating these patients because it is possible to aggravate a preexisting pneumothorax by overaggressive ventilation.

A patient with an acute diaphragmatic hernia seldom requires immediate surgery and anesthesia. The patient should be stabilized with fluids preoperatively. Patients with broken ribs may hypoventilate due to pain. Thus, ventilation should be assisted following intubation. Overaggressive ventilation should be avoided in order to minimize further injury to the adjacent lobes of the lung.

Anesthesia for the patient with chest trauma should include rapid induction and intubation with ventilation assistance. Nitrous oxide should be avoided in patients with free air in the thoracic cavity due to its ability to expand the size of the air space. Nitrous oxide should be used with caution in all patients with thoracic trauma, because its use mandates a decrease in the inspired oxygen concentration. Nitrous oxide should be discontinued in patients that become pale or cyanotic during its use.

Patients with traumatic myocarditis should be converted to normal sinus rhythm prior to anesthesia. Lidocaine, procainamide, and quinidine are three popular antiarrhythmics that can be used. Ventricular arrhythmias that occur during anesthesia can be treated with IV lidocaine (1–2 mg/kg). Halothane should be avoided in patients with ventricular arrhythmias due to its ability to potentiate them. Methoxyflurane, enflurane, or isoflurane can be used with more safety in the patient with ventricular arrhythmias.

Generally, dosages of drugs should be reduced in patients with thoracic trauma, due to reductions in cardiac output. Painful, intractable animals may benefit from narcotic administration. Patients receiving narcotics should be monitored closely for respiratory insufficiency resulting from the drug's respiratory depressant effects.

A useful induction technique for patients following chest trauma includes IV fentanyl citrate–droperidol (Innovar–Vet) (1 ml/20 kg) followed by rapid intubation and anesthetic maintenance with methoxyflurane in oxygen. A small bolus of thiobarbiturate (thiamylal 2–4 mg/kg) may be given to effect and used in dogs that cannot be intubated following fentanyl citrate–droperidol. Cats with thoracic trauma may be induced with a small bolus of ketamine (1–3 mg/kg) then intubated and maintained with inhalation anesthetics.

Gastric Dilation-Volvulus

Gastric dilation-volvulus (GDV) is a pathophysiologically complex disease that requires special attention from the clinician/anesthetist. Gastric dilation-volvulus induces severe cardiopulmonary disturbances including respiratory depression, decreases in cardiac output, and cardiac rhythm disturbances.[9] Decreased cardiac output and respiratory insufficiency lead to hypoperfusion and inadequate oxygenation of peripheral tissues. Hypoperfusion can lead to acid–base disturbances (primarily metabolic acidosis) and shock. Prolonged periods of shock may result in bleeding disorders, including disseminated intravascular coagulopathy.

Preanesthetic supportive care of the patient should begin with decompression of the stomach. The stomach can be deflated via orogastric tube or, if that fails, by percutaneous needle deflation. Deflation combined with the rapid administration of intravenous fluids helps to restore cardiac output. Cardiac arrhythmias usually occur in the postoperative period but may occur at any time. Acid–base status should be assessed and corrected prior to anesthesia. Corticosteroids are indicated if the patient has undergone a period of shock.

Anesthesia for the dog with GDV should emphasize support of ventilation with minimal cardiovascular depression. Ventricular arrhythmias are treated with a lidocaine bolus (1–2 mg/kg) initially, followed with a lidocaine infusion (40–60 μg/kg/min). Lidocaine is a useful agent, because in addition to decreasing ventricular arrhythmias, it may provide some sedation and analgesia, allowing a reduction in dose of other more potent agents. Fluid support of the patient should continue during the surgical procedure. Large volumes of fluid may be required to restore cardiac output.

Dogs with GDV should be induced and intubated rapidly to minimize aspiration of upper airway secretions and vomitus. Intravenous fentanyl citrate-droperidol (1 ml/20 kg) can be used for induction. Alternative techniques include IV diazepam (0.2 mg/kg) followed by IV thiamylal (4–8 mg/kg) administered to effect. Patients with ventricular arrhythmias may be given a reduced dose of thiamylal, supplemented with a bolus of lidocaine (2–4 mg/kg). Etomidate is a new anesthetic induction agent that provides hypnosis with minimal cardiovascular depression. Etomidate is prohibitively expensive and is not approved for use in animals at this time.

Anesthetic levels of inhalation anesthetics usually cause too much depression of the cardiovascular system in dogs with GDV. If the patient does not tolerate inhalation anesthetics, their concentration should be reduced and IV narcotics used to supplement analgesia. Nitrous oxide should not be used due to its ability to enlarge closed gas spaces. Muscle relaxants such as pancuronium (Pavulon 0.02–0.1 mg/kg) may be used to provide muscle relaxation. Respiration must be controlled if muscle relaxants are employed.

Postoperative care of the dog with GDV includes fluid support, acid–base correction, and periodic evaluation for the presence of cardiac dysrhythmias.

Feline Urethral Obstruction

Cats with urethral obstruction can be difficult anesthetiic patients, because they are often dehydrated, acidotic, azotemic, hyperkalemic, hyperphosphatemic, and hypothermic.[2] The severity of these associated metabolic disturbances generally increases with the duration of blockade and is often reflected in the physical appearance of the cat at presentation. Cats that are depressed, weak, and lethargic generally have the most severe derangement.

Anesthesia in the cat with urethral obstruction is divided into two parts: anesthesia for urethral catheterization and anesthesia for perineal urethrostomy. The cat should be rehydrated using normal saline prior to anesthesia. Cats that are weak, depressed, and bradycardic are usually hyperkalemic. Profound bradycardia (less than 60 beats per minute) requires immediate attention. Atropine (0.02 mg/kg) or glycopyrrolate (Robinul 0.01 mg/kg) may decrease vagal tone and increase heart rate. The high serum potassium levels that cause the bradycardia may be acutely lowered by slowly administering IV sodium bicarbonate (1 mEq/kg). Slow boluses of sodium bicarbonate may be repeated at 10-minute intervals. Sodium bicarbonate is effective in correcting metabolic acidosis, in addition to causing an intracellular shift of potassium, thus decreasing extracellular potassium. Response to bicarbonate therapy is monitored by measuring heart rate, ideally using an electrocardiogram. Electrocardiographic signs of hyperkalemia include bradycardia, flattening or absence of the P wave, prolongation of the Q–T interval, and peaking of the T wave. Calcium chloride (10 percent, 1 ml/10 kg) can be given slowly and to effect if sodium bicarbonate is not effective in elevating the heart rate.

Catheterization of the blocked urethra requires only a short period of anesthesia. Comatose cats may not require anesthesia for catheterization. Intravenous ketamine (1–2 mg/kg) administered to effect is a good choice in cats that require anesthesia for catheterization. The diuresis that occurs after the relief of obstruction allows elimination of a major part of the ketamine administered. Some clinicians prefer IV thiamylal sodium (2–6 mg/kg) administered slowly and to effect, because thiamylal offers a greater degree of muscle relaxation than ketamine, facilitating catheterization. The author prefers ketamine, because it produces less deleterious cardiopulmonary side effects than thiamylal. Muscle relaxation may be increased with ketamine by using diazepam (0.2 mg/kg) in combination. Xylazine should not be used in cats with urethral obstruction, because it potentiates bradycardia and ventricular arrhythmias.

Anesthesia for perineal urethrostomy should not be attempted until the obstruction has been relieved and the cat's metabolic status is returned to normal. Perineal urethrostomy is only an emergency procedure if a catheter cannot be passed or a cystocentesis cannot be done. Perineal urethrostomy cats are preanesthetized with IV diazepam (0.2 mg/kg). General anesthesia is introduced with either ketamine (1–2 mg/kg) or thiamylal (4–8 mg/kg) given IV slowly and to effect. Halothane is not recommended in the cat with cardiac rhythm abnormalities. Methoxyflurane-induced renal failure has not been demonstrated in animals, although methoxyflurane has been incriminated as a cause of postoperative renal failure in humans. Isoflurane, a newer inhalation anesthetic, would be ideal for use but is cost prohibitive. Stabilized cats who have their metabolic derangements corrected prior to surgery do not pose a particular anesthetic challenge, thus, either halothane or methoxyflurane may be safely used.

Caesarean Section

Anesthesia for Caesarean section has been a subject of discussion since the time of the Roman Empire. Many anesthetic plans have been proposed and discussed in the literature. This discussion will center on the physiology of pregnancy and fetal life and the principles of passage of drugs across the placenta.

The pregnant animal increases its blood volume, cardiac output, and oxygen consumption during pregnancy in order to meet the demands of the fetus.[10] Resting lung volumes and overall lung capacity decrease as the abdomen increases in size due to cranial displacement of the diaphragm. Liver function is decreased, while renal plasma flow and glomerular filtration are increased during pregnancy.[3]

Tremendous expenditures of energy occur as the female enters labor. The parturient often refuses food and often will refuse to drink. Prolonged labor may result in exhaustion (hypoglycemia), dehydration, and hypocalcemia. Increased abdominal pressure during labor may induce regurgitation. Food and water should be withheld to minimize the quantity of stomach contents, if surgery is anticipated.

The fetus receives all oxygen and nutrients from its mother. The fetal blood pH is lower than maternal pH, which promotes the release of oxygen to fetal tissues.[6] Fetal hemoglobin has a greater affinity for oxygen than maternal hemoglobin. During labor, fetal stress parallels maternal stress, thus an exhausted female often delivers weak newborns.

Maternal hydration should be restored prior to anesthesia. Glucose and calcium solutions should be administered prior to anesthesia if the patient is exhausted or hypocalcemic. Clipping of hair and the initial surgical scrub should be performed before any anesthetic drugs are given. It is important to minimize the time between administration of drugs and delivery of the fetus. Anesthetic principles for Caesarean section include oxygenation of the mother and protection of the airway. Analgesia and restraint of the mother must be provided while producing minimal fetal depression. Anesthetic techniques for the Caesarean section vary according to the species, the facility, the technical help available, and the ability of the surgeon-anesthetist.

Epidural anesthesia is best for the fetus. Cranial epidural anesthesia (injection at the lumbosacral space) provides regional anesthesia for the dam and good muscle relaxation of the abdominal wall, while minimally depressing the fetus.[6] Local anesthetics, when absorbed into the systemic circulation, do cross the placental barrier, but at low levels. Fluids should be administered prior to and during epidural anesthesia because the epidural anesthetic will induce hypotension due to loss of sympathetic tone in the part of the body that is desensitized. Tranquilization of the dam may be required in order to position her for surgery. Subcutaneous administration of acetylpromazine (PromAce 0.1–0.2 mg/kg) or lenperone (Elanone-V 0.1–0.2 mg/kg) can be used for tranquilization. Both acetylpromazine and lenperone will cross the placenta and depress the fetus, therefore doses should be kept to a minimum. Duration of epidural anesthesia is 60–90 minutes. Time to peak anesthesia post-injection may be up to 20 minutes. Oxygen may be supplemented by face mask during epidural anesthesia.

Time from induction to removal of the fetus is of utmost importance if general anesthesia is used. The animal should be intubated to maximize control of the dam's airway. Drugs that depress the dam will cause fetal depression. Respiratory depression must be minimized so respiration can be stimulated in the newborn.

Narcotics are useful for Caesarean section in the dog. Although narcotics are respiratory depressants and cross the placental barrier, their effects are reversible by administering naloxone to the puppies. Single boluses of ultra-short-acting thiobarbiturates can be used for short-duration anesthesia or induction to general anesthesia. Pentobarbital or multiple doses of thiobarbiturates should not be administered if viable newborns are anticipated. Xylazine should be avoided because it is a profound cardiopulmonary depressant. Cats maybe anesthetized with IV ketamine (1–2 mg/kg).

Maintenance of anesthesia can be accomplished by many techniques. Halothane depresses the respiratory centers the least, when compared with the inhalation agents currently in use. Halothane may be combined with nitrous oxide. Newborns delivered with halothane anesthesia are depressed, but once stimulated to breathe, recover rapidly. Halothane causes increased uterine bleeding in women and may retard involution of the uterus. Due to differences in placentation excessive bleeding is less of a problem in veterinary medicine. Methoxyflurane is a greater respiratory depressant and is eliminated more slowly, thus it should only be used in very low concentrations. Ideally, the fetus should be removed prior to the initiation of inhalation anesthesia, while the dam is under the effect of the induction agent. Narcotics given in intermittent boluses can be used to continue anesthesia during Caesarean section. If fentanyl citrate–droperidol is used to induce anesthesia, fentanyl citrate (0.001–0.003 mg/kg) can be used to maintain analgesia. Fentanyl citrate is given in intermittent boluses as needed, which is usually every 20 minutes. Narcotics produce minimal cardiovascular depression but may cause bradycardia. Bradycardia due to narcotic administration is responsive to anticholinergic drug administration. Respiratory depression in the newborn can be reversed by the administration of naloxone into the umbilical vein.

Muscle relaxants have been advocated for use in Caesarean section.[5] Due to their structure, muscle relaxants cross the placental barrier very slowly, in minimal quantity. Practically speaking, muscle relaxants do not affect the fetus when administered to the dam. Disadvantages of using muscle relaxants include postoperative weakness in the bitch and requirement of positive pressure ventilation because the animal cannot breathe. Muscle relaxants provide no analgesia, so analgesia must be provided using narcotics or thiobarbiturates.

Following delivery, the airway of the neonate should be cleared and respiration stimulation by rubbing the thorax and abdomen with a dry towel. If respiration does not begin, doxapram (Dopram) can be administered sublingually or injected via the umbilical vein. Naloxone can be given to the neonate via the umbilicus if the dam had been given narcotics. The neonate should be dried and warmed in an oxygen-enriched atmosphere. A fish tank or anesthetic induction chamber can be used to provide an enriched oxygen atmosphere. Neonates should be placed with the mother when she has fully recovered from anesthesia. Hydration of the mother should be maintained to allow for adequate milk production.

REFERENCES

1. Albrecht DT, Blakely CL: Anesthetic mortality: A five year survey of records of the Angell Memorial Hospital. J Am Vet Med Assoc 119:429, 1951
2. Burrows CF, Bovee KC: Characterization and treatment of acid–base and renal defects due to urethral obstruction in cats. Am Vet Med Assoc 172:801, 1978
3. Cohen SE: Why is the pregnant patient different? American Society of Anesthesiologists Refresher Course lectures. New Orleans, LA 1981
4. Cornelius CE: Liver Function in Clinical Biochemistry of Domestic Animals. 3rd Ed. Academic Press, San Diego, 1980
5. Dodman NH: Anaesthesia for Caesarean section in the dog and cat: A review. J Small Anim Pract 20:449, 1979

6. Hartsfield SM: Obstetrical anesthesia in small animals. California Veterinarian, p. 18. September, 1979
7. MacIntire DK, Snider TG: Cardiac arrhythmias associated with multiple trauma in dogs. J Am Vet Med Assoc 184:541, 1984
8. Nagel ML, Muir WW, Nguyen K: Comparison of the cardiopulmonary effects of etomidate and thiamylal in dogs. Am J Vet Res 40:193 1979
9. Orton EC, Muir WW: Hemodynamics during experimental gastric dilatation-volvulus in dogs. Am J Vet Res 44:1512, 1983
10. Pedersen H, Finster M: Anesthetic risk in the pregnant surgical patient. Anesthesiology 5:439, 1979
11. Rawlings CA, Kolata RJ: Cardiopulmonary effects of thiopental/lidocaine combination during anesthetic induction in the dog. Am J Vet Res 44:144, 1983
12. Robinson NE and Gillespie JR: Pulmonary diffusing capacity and capillary blood volume in aging dogs. J Appl Physiol 48:647, 1975
13. Smith AL: Barbiturate protection in primate cerebral ischemia. Abstracts of Scientific Papers. American Society of Anesthesiologists Annual Meeting p. 143, 1974
14. Tamas P, Paddleford RR, Krahwinkel DJ: Incidence of thoracic trauma in conjunction with limb fractures following motor vehicle accidents in dogs and cats. Scientific meetings, American College of Veterinary Anesthesiologists, Atlanta, GA, 1983
15. Wilkinson L: Anesthesia for intracranial surgery with particular reference to surgery for neoplasms. Adv Neurol 15:253, 1975

4 Radiologic Considerations for the Emergency Patient

Norman Ackerman
Crispin P. Spencer

CLINICAL INDICATIONS

The often repeated statement that "an animal should not be permitted to die in radiology" emphasizes the considerations in evaluating the emergency patient. There are only a few situations in which radiology is the only method of confirming the diagnosis of a life-threatening emergency. Radiography should be postponed if the expected benefits do not exceed the risks associated with patient restraint and manipulation; and a compromise between the clinician's desire for information and the danger to the patient is often necessary.

Analgesics, tranquilizers, and/or narcotics should be used when possible. These permit restraint of the patient without struggling or added stress.

Although two radiographic views are usually considered necessary, the patient's condition may preclude obtaining more than one view. Lateral views are generally more convenient, quicker, less stressful, and they do not require patient manipulation into an uncomfortable or awkward position. In certain instances, a dorsoventral view may be more convenient. Horizontal beam or standing views are useful when the patient resents lateral, sternal, or dorsal recumbancy. Manipulation and restraint should be minimized so that the patient's condition is not aggravated.

Each radiography room should be equipped with the drugs and equipment necessary for resuscitation or treatment of an emergency patient. If the individuals radiographing the patient are different from those who initially treated the case, communication regarding the patient's status and possible diagnosis is critical.

SKULL

The skull is a rather complex structure and, in most instances, careful symmetrical positioning and multiple radiographic views are required for critical evaluation and accurate interpretation. Compression or depression fractures may require immediate radiographic evaluation and surgical intervention; however, if the patient can be anesthetized for surgery, the required radiographs can and should be obtained at the same time.

Skull fractures are recognized by the presence of a radiolucent fracture line, the increased density resulting from overlapping of fragments, or the skull deformity associated with fragment displacement. Vascular channels or open sutures may be mistaken for fractures; however, these structures are usually symmetrical and can be recognized by their location. In order to be certain that a fracture, rather than a normal suture, is present, a widened or malaligned suture line must be identified. Fractures should be evaluated for involvement of the teeth, osseous bulla, temporomandibular or atlanto-occipital joints. Often, only a portion of the fracture line is evident on a single radiographic view and several oblique views are necessary for complete evaluation.

Dislocation of the temporomandibular joint is readily recognized if the animal is positioned properly. Comparison of the right and left sides is essential. Careful examination for fractures of the condylar, angular, or retroglenoid processes is important. These may be small and easily overlooked and can complicate reduction of the dislocation.[11]

SPINE

Fracture, dislocation, and disc disease are the most frequent conditions seen as radiologic emergencies. Marked displacement of vertebrae or fracture fragments is easily identified, and a single lateral radiograph is often sufficient, but in some cases may be misleading. Articular facet fractures, minimally displaced or slightly malaligned vertebrae, can be more difficult to identify. Patient manipulation or struggling may cause further displacement of an incomplete or slightly displaced fracture or luxation; for that reason, general anesthesia is preferred for radiographic evaluation. The patient should be kept in lateral recumbancy if dorsal recumbant radiographs are needed. Horizontal beam radiographs may be used in lieu of dorsal recumbant views; however, they are usually of poor quality due to a loss of radiographic detail.

Vertebral body fractures may be compression fractures and, as such, difficult to detect. Shortening of the vertebral segment or altered bony trabecular patterns may be the initial clues to the diagnosis.[9] Pathologic fractures may present as acute emergencies with or without a history of prior trauma. All fractures must be carefully examined for evidence of bone destruction or proliferation which indicates an underlying or preexisting metabolic, infectious, or neoplastic disease resulting in a pathologic fracture.

Malalignment following dislocation may be slight and easily overlooked.[9] An abrupt change in angulation of the vertebral segments, narrowing or widening of the intervertebral disc space or vertebral joint space may be clues to the presence of a luxation. Small fracture fragments may occur around the articular facets or at the margins of the vertebral bodies (Fig. 4-1).

Displacement or malalignment of vertebral segments greater than 50 percent of the spinal canal width is usually indicative of severe spinal cord injury. This is influenced by the level at which the fracture or dislocation occurred and also the presence or absence of an intact dorsal arch. Dorsal arch fractures can permit cord displacement without cord compression.

A congenital anomaly such as absence or hypoplasia of the dens may allow vertebral segment displacement with minimal trauma. This anomaly should be easily recognized, especially in those toy breeds in which it is usually seen. Manipulation of the head and neck must be cautiously performed if this diagnosis is suspected. An increased distance between the atlas and axis as the head is flexed, with or without a hypoplastic, absent, or fractured odontoid process will be observed.

Intervertebral disc disease often presents as an emergency. The most common radiographic findings are disc space narrowing; increased density, altered shape, or decreased size of the intervertebral foramen; overlapping of the articular facets (decreased interarcuate space); or mineralized density within the spinal canal. It is a serious mistake to evaluate disc disease in an unanesthetized or poorly positioned patient. Artifacts resulting from failure to stretch the spine, rotation, or angulation of the spine or off-centering of the x-ray beam can mimic or obscure radiographic evidence of disc disease. When clinical and neurologic signs do not fit the radiographic lesion, a myelogram is essential if surgery is contemplated.

THORAX

Most thoracic emergencies involve patients who exhibit some degree of respiratory distress; therefore, restraint should be minimized. The initial radiograph (either a lateral or a dorsoventral view) should be exposed with the patient positioned comfortably and minimally restrained. After this radiograph is evaluated and the patient's condition is assessed, a decision can be made regarding the need for additional views. If the patient cannot be positioned in sternal or dorsal recumbancy, the lungs can be evaluated using both right and left lateral recumbant views.[10]

The bony thorax should be examined for rib or vertebral fractures (Fig. 4-1). Multiple segmental rib fractures can create an unstable thoracic wall (i.e., flail chest) that collapses on inspiration and compromises respiration. A dis-

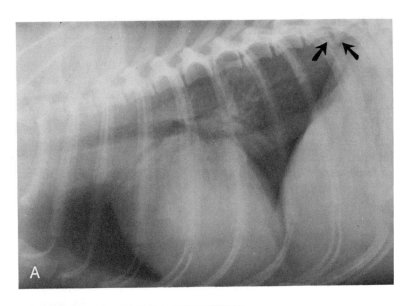

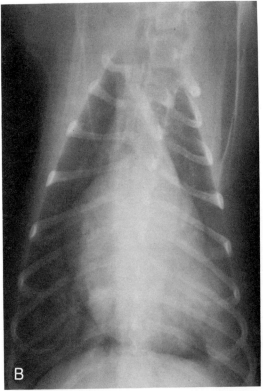

Fig. 4-1. Lateral (A) and dorsoventral (B) thoracic radiographs of a 1-year-old poodle presented after being hit by a car. A left shoulder luxation and brachial plexus avulsion were suspected due to loss of reflexes and pain in the left forelimb. An increased pulmonary density is evident in the left caudal lung lobe. This is most likely the result of pulmonary contusions or hemorrhage. Careful systematic evaluation of the radiograph revealed a fracture luxation at T10–11 (arrows) with ventral displacement of T-11. Failure to evaluate the radiograph thoroughly would have delayed the diagnosis of this lesion and might have compromised the dog's condition.

placed rib may traumatize the lung if anesthesia or positive pressure ventilation become necessary; therefore, it should not be overlooked.[9]

Acute respiratory distress may result from pathology within the lung or within the pleural space. These can be differentiated radiographically and, in many cases, a specific etiology can be recognized.

The presence of a fluid infiltrate within the lung can be identified because of the pattern that results. This has been described as a reticular or nodular interstitial pattern or an alveolar pattern that tends to coalesce and produce branching, radiolucent, air bronchograms. The presence of either of these patterns indicates that the fluid density is within the lung (Fig. 4-2). Interstitial or alveolar fluid may be blood, edema, or pus. The pattern may be the same; however, the distribution of the densities within the various lung lobes will be a clue to the probable diagnosis.[6]

Localized alveolar or interstitial fluid densities may occur as a result of bacterial pneumonia, aspiration pneumonia, pulmonary contusion or hemorrhage, or thromboembolic disease. Generalized alveolar or interstitial fluid density may be classified into cardiogenic and noncardiogenic causes. The size of the cardiac silhouette is an important clue in distinguishing between these two classifications: left heart enlargement usually accompanies cardiogenic, and right heart enlargement accompanies noncardiogenic pulmonary edema. Noncardiogenic pulmonary edemas occur postictally, post-expansionally, after electric shock, cranial trauma, severe allergic reactions, and exposure to some toxins, and under many other conditions.

Dyspnea may also result from accumulation of fluid, masses, viscera, or air in the pleural space. Pleural fluid will be recognized because it separates the lungs from the lateral thoracic wall, outlines the individual lung lobes, obliterates the cardiac silhouette and diaphragm, and causes the cranial and/ or caudal mediastinum to widen[4] (Fig. 4-3). Only rarely it is possible to determine the nature of the pleural fluid, based on radiographic signs. A thoracocentesis is usually required. Pleural masses and loculated or trapped pleural fluid may produce similar radiographic appearances. Displacement of the lung and mediastinal structures away from the homogenous soft tissue density will occur in both instances. Rib involvement (either bony proliferation or destruction) or extension of the soft tissue density through an intercostal space to produce an external soft tissue swelling indicates a pleural mass. Diaphragmatic hernia can usually be recognized because of the interruption in diaphragmatic outline and the presence of gas or ingesta-filled bowel within the pleural space; however, pleural effusion may result, especially if a liver lobe becomes trapped. This may be difficult to determine without complete fluid removal and positional views. Lung lobe torsion also causes pleural fluid, therefore all lung lobes should be identified when pleural fluid is present. Pleural fluid usually becomes distributed evenly throughout the pleural space. Accumulation of fluid in a localized area or failure of fluid to move with changes in the patient's position may indicate an abnormality such as pneumonia, abscess, tumor, or torsion of the lung lobe normally found in that location. Radiographs obtained following fluid removal will identify the pulmonary abnormality.

(*Text continues on page 69*)

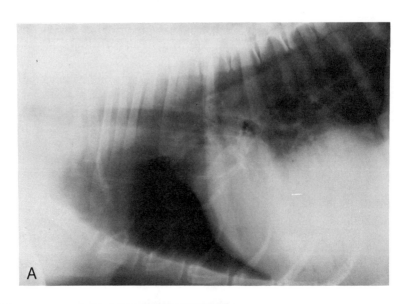

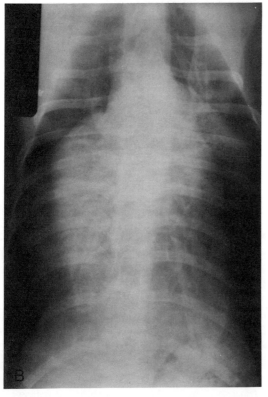

Fig. 4-2. Lateral (A) and dorsoventral (B) radiographs of a 2-year-old Great Dane presented with anorexia, depression, dyspnea, and a cough of 1 week duration. A large soft tissue density is evident in the ventral caudal thorax, obliterating the cardiac silhouette and diaphragm. Air bronchograms are visible within this density, indicating that the lung is involved and the alveoli contain fluid. This is important in ruling out diaphragmatic hernia or a pleural mass in this case. The bacterial pneumonia that involves the accessory and ventral portion of the left caudal lung lobe responded to antibiotics within 12 days.

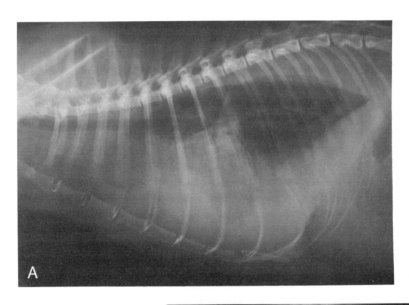

Fig. 4-3. Lateral (A) and ventrodorsal (B) radiographs of a two-year-old feline presented with dyspnea and weight loss and dull respiratory sounds. The cardiac silhouette and diaphragm are obscured and the lung lobes are outlined and separated from the thoracic wall by a soft tissue density. These findings are indicative of pleural fluid.

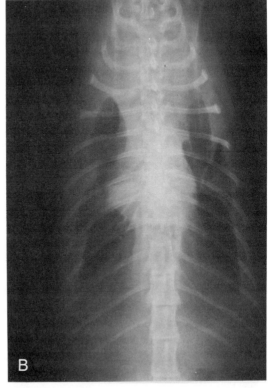

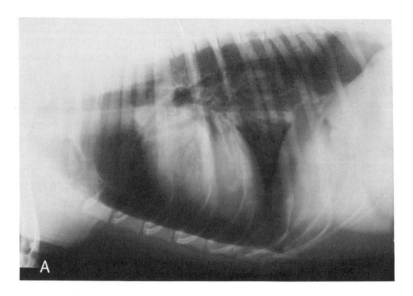

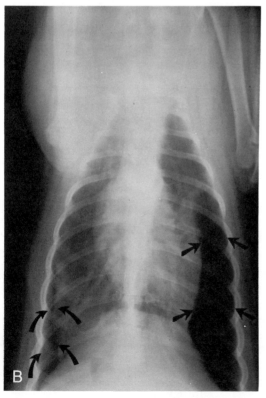

Fig. 4-4. Lateral (A) and dorsoventral (B) radiographs of a 2-year-old mixed breed dog presented after having been hit by a car. The cardiac silhouette is separated from the sternum, and the lungs are collapsed and separated from the thoracic wall by an air density. There is a greater volume of pleural air on the left side (straight arrows) than on the right side (curved arrows). The uneven air accumulation indicates the presence of pathology in the left lung that interferes with its inflation. After removal of the pleural air, pulmonary infiltrate secondary to pulmonary contusion and several intrapulmonary hematomas were identified in the left lung.

Air within the pleural space will outline the lung lobe margins and separate the heart from the sternum (Fig. 4-4). Careful examination of the radiolucent areas will demonstrate the absence of pulmonary vessels. Separation of the heart from the sternum is a sign of mediastinal shift toward the dependent side and should be interpreted cautiously since it can be produced by conditions other than pneumothorax. Tension pneumothorax, which occurs when air is forced into the pleural space on inspiration but cannot escape on expiration, is accompanied by severe pulmonary collapse, with large amounts of free pleural gas. The parietal pleural surface may appear scalloped, because of high pressures within the pleural space. The diaphragm will be displaced caudally. Unilateral tension pneumothorax will cause a mediastinal shift toward the unaffected side. Air within the pleural space usually moves freely with changes in patient position and becomes distributed evenly within both right and left pleural cavities. Uneven distribution of pleural air with more severe collapse of one lung lobe is indicative of disease within the densest lung lobe (Fig. 4-4). This will become more obvious after the air is removed.[3,9] There is a poor correlation between the amount of pleural air seen radiographically and the animal's clinical signs; when tension pneumothorax is identified, immediate removal of air is indicated.

Tracheal injury or foreign body may produce a sudden onset of respiratory distress. The alteration in tracheal shape or presence of a tissue density within the trachea should not be missed if the trachea is carefully examined.[5] Tracheal perforation may produce pneumomediastinum or pneumothorax. Pneumomediastinum may be recognized because of the air outlining the soft tissue structures within the mediastinum. The air may also migrate subcutaneously or caudally along the aorta into the retroperitoneal space. Although pneumomediastinum may progress to pneumothorax, the reverse does not occur.[5,9]

ABDOMEN

As with the thorax, it is often necessary to evaluate a lateral radiograph first and decide if additional views are needed and can be obtained without danger to the patient.

Fluid in the peritoneal cavity (i.e., blood, pus, transudate, or urine) results in the loss of abdominal visceral detail. Young or emaciated animals, which lack abdominal fat, do not have good visceral detail; therefore, recognizing abdominal fluid in these patients is difficult.[7] A paracentesis is necessary to determine the nature of the abdominal fluid. If urine is obtained from the paracentesis, a renal, ureteral, bladder, or urethral tear may be present. Urethral and bladder rupture should be evaluated by positive contrast cystourethrography. Urine and blood may accumulate in the retroperitoneal space; in some cases of ureteral or renal trauma, a paracentesis can be negative. Pneumocystography is not satisfactory; although the presence of bladder rupture can be confirmed, the site of the rupture is not outlined. If these studies are negative, an excretory urogram should be performed.

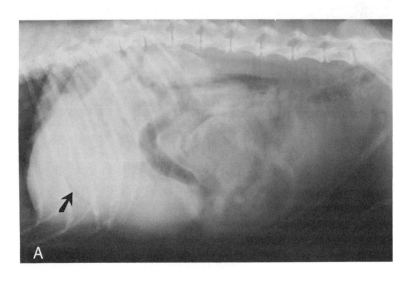

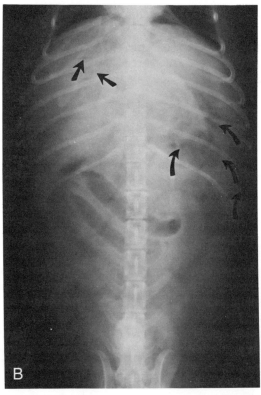

Fig. 4-5. Lateral (A) and ventrodorsal (B) abdominal radiographs of a 10-year-old sheltie presented with a history of depression, vomiting, and anorexia for 24 hours. The abdomen was not painful, and the dog's temperature was 99°F. Abdominal visceral detail is poor, especially in the midventral abdomen. Small gas bubbles are evident in the splenic area on the ventrodorsal radiograph (curved arrows), and linear gas accumulations are evident between the stomach and liver on the lateral radiograph and between liver lobes on the ventrodorsal radiograph (straight arrows). A horizontal beam right lateral recumbant radiograph

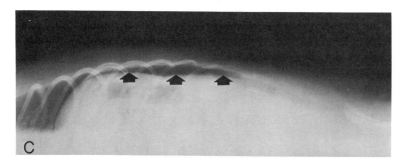

Fig. 4-5. (*continued*)   (C) was obtained, and free air is visible beneath the left thoracic wall (wide arrows). The radiographic changes are indicative of bowel rupture with peritonitis. A perforated duodenal ulcer was found at laparotomy.

Loss of abdominal visceral detail may be localized due to peritonitis, pancreatitis, or carcinomatosis.[7] The location of the fluid density should be correlated with the normal structures in that portion of the abdomen. Peritoneal lavage may be necessary to identify the cause of the fluid accumulation, since small amounts of fluid or cellular infiltrate may be present, and fluid may not be obtained by a needle paracentesis.

Peritoneal air indicates a penetrating wound, a ruptured viscus, previous surgery, or previous paracentesis.[7] Spontaneous pneumoperitoneum has been described following gastric dilatation-volvulus. In one case, bacterial infection with a gas-producing organism was suggested as the cause of the peritoneal air since gastric perforation was not identified. A rupture of the stomach at the gastroesophageal junction was identified in another case.[8] Peritoneal gas usually accumulates in the highest portion of the abdomen. In lateral recumbancy, this is caudal to the dorsal portion of the diaphragm between the liver lobes. If peritoneal gas is suspected, a horizontal beam radiograph can be used to confirm the diagnosis.[7,12] Left lateral recumbancy is preferred, since confusion with the gastric air bubble can be avoided (Fig. 4-5). Peritoneal air may be present as long as 30 days after surgery. This must be considered when evaluating the abdominal radiographs of those patients with recent surgery. Gastrointestinal contrast radiography using micronized barium sulfate is contraindicated if bowel perforation is suspected. A water soluble contrast agent (Oral Hypaque) should be used.

Gastric dilatation-volvulus and partial gastric dilatation-volvulus may be identified radiographically.[7] The acute distress and clinical signs in complete volvulus usually lead to a diagnosis without radiography. Radiographically, a gastric compartmentalization resulting from the stomach folding on itself has been described.[7] The pyloric and cardiac-fundic portion of the stomach can usually be recognized because of their size and shape, even when distended. Displacement of the pylorus dorsally and to the left can be detected radiographically in complete and partial gastric dilatation-volvulus. If partial gastric dilatation-volvulus is suspected, four views of the cranial abdomen should be obtained (i.e., right and left lateral recumbant, ventrodorsal and dorsoventral). The position of the gastric fluid and air within the stomach as the patient is manipulated indicates the position of the stomach within the abdomen. Micronized colloidal barium sulfate (Colibar-V) may be used to help identify the stomach, but this is rarely necessary. Splenomegaly, esophageal dilatation, compression of the caudal vena cava, and ileus may also be observed.

Intestinal obstruction may be classified as high or low, and complete or incomplete.[7] The radiographic changes observed vary according to the nature of the obstruction. High intestinal obstruction (i.e., proximal to the jejunum) results in gastric and some duodenal distension. Reverse peristalsis allows fluid or ingesta to return to the stomach, and the animal will vomit, eliminating most of the material. The stomach usually remains distended, despite the recurrent vomiting. Low obstruction (i.e., jejunum and ileum) produces distention of the small intestine with fluid, gas, or food material. The distension of the intestine (ileus) can be recognized radiographically when the diameter of the small intestine approaches or exceeds the diameter of the large intestine. Intestinal obstruction may be mechanical (due to foreign objects, strictures, tumors, granulomas, intussusception, etc.) or paralytic (due to drugs, neurogenic causes, vascular compromise, pain, etc.), however, in many cases, a definite cause cannot be determined radiographically. Although horizontal beam radiographs have been recommended, they are usually not helpful in distinguishing between mechanical and paralytic obstruction.

If the obstruction is incomplete or recent, some food, fluid, or gas may still be present distal to the site of the obstruction; in most complete obstructions, the bowel distal to the site of the obstruction will be empty. Fluid or gas may get past an incomplete obstruction, while solid material such as bone or solid food will accumulate. This may result in distention of the intestine with a granular, dense material. When the obstruction is complete, a large amount of gas and fluid accumulates and distends the intestinal loops. Gastrointestinal contrast studies are not indicated, if complete obstruction can be recognized on the plain films. In most cases, the patient will vomit the contrast material or the contrast will remain in the stomach, never reaching the obstruction. Delaying surgery to perform a contrast study under these circumstances is contraindicated. If an incomplete obstruction can be identified based on plain film findings, a gastrointestinal contrast study is not necessary. If the diagnosis is uncertain, or more information regarding the exact cause, extent, and location of the partial obstruction is needed by the surgeon or owner before surgery is performed, a gastrointestinal contrast study should be performed. Micronized barium sulfate (Colibar-V) should be used rather than iodinated contrast agents for the study, because of the superior anatomic detail that micronized barium produces. Although the iodine-containing contrast agents transit the gastrointestinal tract more rapidly, they do not delineate structures very well, and, because of their hypertonicity, they may dehydrate the patient.

Splenic torsion is a rare cause of acute abdominal distress. The enlarged spleen with rounded edges may be recognized in the right anterior abdomen. A variable amount of peritoneal fluid may be present, obscuring visceral detail.

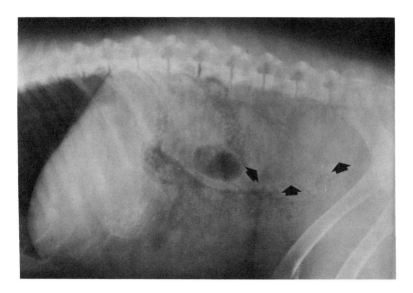

Fig. 4-6. Lateral abdominal radiograph of a 5-month-old mixed breed dog presented 1 hour after having been hit by a car. The colon is displaced ventrally and the sublumbar (retroperitoneal) area is dense and indistinct ventral to L-5, -6, and -7 (arrows). These findings are indicative of sublumbar fluid accumulation. This is most likely hemorrhage associated with the dog's pelvic fractures; however, urine accumulation from a ureteral tear would produce similar radiographic changes.

The shape of the stomach may be distorted due to twisting of the gastrosplenic ligament.[7]

Uterine enlargement associated with pyometra may present as an abdominal emergency. The fluid-distended tubular loops that displace the small intestines cranially and dorsally can be recognized on abdominal radiographs. An enlarged uterus resulting from pyometra may be confused with a gravid uterus during an interval from 30 to 42 days after conception. Before 30 days, the ampullation or segmentation of the pregnant uterus can be recognized, and after 42 days, mineralization of the feti can be detected. This helps to differentiate pregnancy from pyometra.[1,7]

Retroperitoneal fluid or swelling may be detected radiographically by swelling in the sublumbar area or by ventral displacement of the colon.[1,9] Retroperitoneal hemorrhage often results from pelvic trauma (Fig. 4-6). Excretory urography is required if renal or ureteral trauma is suspected.

EXTREMITIES

Trauma is a common cause of emergencies involving the long bones and joints. Radiographic evaluation is important in treatment planning and prognosis; however, the patient should be stabilized before radiographs are obtained.

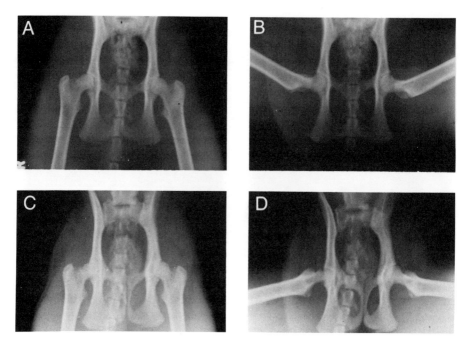

Fig. 4-7. Ventrodorsal pelvic radiographs of a 4-month-old cat presented with a right rear limb lameness thought to be secondary to trauma. The initial radiographs (A and B) were interpreted as normal. Additional radiographs (C and D) obtained 1 week later demonstrate the right femoral capital epiphyseal fracture.

Despite a history of trauma, all fractures should be evaluated for altered bone density which indicates that a preexisting disease produced a pathologic fracture. Many bone diseases produce few clinical signs until a pathologic fracture occurs.

All fractures must be carefully evaluated, utilizing two projections made at right angles to each other and including the joints proximal and distal to the fracture. The fracture fragments should be examined closely for fissures or cracks that might complicate the repair. The soft tissues in the fracture area should be examined for the presence of subcutaneous air that indicates an open wound. In immature animals with open physes or incompletely mineralized bones, comparison radiographs of the normal limb are extremely valuable in assessing the nature and extent of the bony or ligamentous injury. Physeal trauma or incomplete fractures may not be recognized initially. If clinical evidence of pain and lameness persists, a repeat radiographic evaluation is essential to evaluate the growth plate or fracture site (Fig. 4-7).

Stress or weight bearing radiographs are useful in assessing the site and nature of a joint or ligamentous injury. These views are usually taken in addition to the standard two views and will confirm the extent of ligamentous injury already detected by physical examination of the limb.[2]

CONCLUSION

There are few indications for emergency radiography. The stress of manipulating and restraining the patient must be minimized and the patient's safety should be more important than a textbook quality radiograph. Some of the more commonly encountered emergency conditions in which radiographic evaluation is helpful have been reviewed in this chapter.

REFERENCES

1. Ackerman N: Radiology of Urogenital Diseases in Dogs and Cats. Venture Press, Davis, 1983
2. Farrow CS: Carpal sprain injury in the dog. Vet Radiol 180:38, 1977
3. Myer W: Pneumothorax: a radiography review. Vet Radiol 19:12, 1978
4. Myer W: Radiography review: pleural effusion. Vet Radiol 19:75, 1978
5. Myer W: Radiography review: the mediastinum. Vet Radiol 19:197, 1978
6. Myer W: Radiography review: the alveolar pattern of pulmonary disease. Vet Radiol 20:10, 1979
7. O'Brien TR: Radiographic Diagnosis of Abdominal Disorders in the Dog and Cat. Covell Park Vet Co, Davis, 1982
8. Probst CW, Bright RM, Ackerman N et al: Spontaneous pneumoperitoneum subsequent to gastric volvulus in two dogs. Vet Radiol 25:37, 1984
9. Spencer CP and Ackerman, N: Thoracic and abdominal radiography of the trauma patient. Vet Clin North Am 10:541, 1980
10. Spencer CP, Ackerman, N, Burt, JK: The canine lateral thoracic radiograph. Vet Radiol 22:262, 1981
11. Ticer JW, Spencer, CP: Injury of the feline temporomandibular joint: radiographic signs. Vet Radiol 19:146, 1978
12. Walker MA: Horizontal beam radiography: diagnostic aid for trauma of the abdomen and extremities. Am Anim Hosp Assoc Proceedings 2:254, 1975

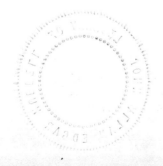

5 | General Principles of Early Wound Care

Curtis W. Probst

A wound is defined as a bodily injury caused by trauma, with disruption of the normal continuity of structures. The sources of trauma include: simple lacerations; automobile accidents; bite wounds; gunshot wounds; burns; incorrect application of bandages, casts, and splints; decubital ulcers; perivascular injection of hypertonic drugs[34]; and the surgeon's knife. The degree of tissue damage resulting from such trauma will vary, but the principles of wound management remain the same.

There are two types of wounds, i.e., penetrating and non-penetrating. Nonpenetrating wounds are caused by blunt forces that do not break the skin. Such forces cause kinetic energy to dissipate throughout the underlying tissues, resulting in varying degrees of trauma. Nonpenetrating wounds can have severely damaged deep tissues with little or no external evidence of trauma.

Penetrating, or open wounds are accompanied by varying degrees of contamination and tissue damage, depending on the manner in which the wounds were sustained. A laceration from a piece of glass, for example, will likely have less tissue damage and bacterial inoculation than a wound resulting from a dog bite.

CLASSIFICATION OF OPEN WOUNDS

The early time period following wounding is called the "golden period." This period is variable in length, and it is generally considered to extend for 6 hours after the time of injury. During this "golden period" wounds may be decontaminated by debridement and lavage; however, after this period, bacteria have begun invading beyond the wound margins. Three hours after wounding is regarded as a critical time, since it has been found that bacterial numbers are approaching the dangerous level of greater than 10^5 bacteria per gram of tissue.[33]

Open wounds can be categorized into three classes, depending on the progression of infection.[7] A class 1 wound is 0 to 6 hours old, and little bacterial multiplication has taken place. A class 2 wound is 6 to 12 hours old, during which time bacteria have begun dividing but have not invaded beyond the wound margins. A class 3 wound is over 12 hours old and is usually infected.

The time division in wound classification is arbitrary and will be modified by the nature of the wound, the circumstances of wounding, and the integrity of local blood supply.[7] The surgeon must recognize that the time between wounding and definitive treatment is less important when compared to the effectiveness of local defense mechanisms and the virulence and number of bacteria inoculated.[9,10,13,18,33,34]

Management of the Open Wound

Suturing a wound within a few hours of injury is termed *primary closure*. If suturing a wound is initially postponed, but is performed before granulation tissue appears, it is termed *delayed primary closure*. Suturing wounds after granulation tissue has appeared is called *secondary closure*. Second intention healing, or, more appropriately termed, *healing by contraction and epithelization*, usually occurs in wounds that are not sutured.[9,33]

Wound healing following suture closure is the goal of wound management.[4,9] Primary wound closure is indicated if there is little chance of wound infection and dehiscence after closure. Whether a wound becomes infected depends on the effectiveness of local defense mechanisms and the extent of bacterial contamination.[9,13,14,18,30,33,34] The circumstances of wounding, the initial wound care, and the definitive wound management will influence these two factors. Local tissue resistance to infection is primarily a function of blood supply, which is often compromised in wounds that have sustained crushing, bruising or tearing of tissue. Overzealous first-aid attempts may needlessly contaminate wounds before the veterinarian sees them.[33,34] Necrotic tissue, soil, hair, or other foreign material in the wound will significantly decrease tissue resistance to infection.[9,33,34] Adequate wound debridement to minimize the chances of wound infection is imperative in these cases.

The decision to close a wound primarily should be based on the assessment of the integrity of local tissue defense mechanisms and estimation of the number and virulence of bacteria present, not merely upon the time interval since wounding.[9,33,34] Wounds with severe tissue trauma and heavy bacterial and foreign material contamination are not suitable for closure, even immediately after wounding. Conversely, wounds with minimal tissue damage, intact blood supply, and small bacterial contamination may be safely closed even after the "golden period."[9] If any doubt exists whether or not a wound should be closed primarily, it should be managed as an open wound until a more accurate wound assessment can be made.

Assessment of the Animal

Before beginning definitive wound treatment, the animal must be carefully examined for concurrent injuries. Depending on the manner in which the wound was sustained, the animal may present with a variety of other problems, including pneumothorax, hypovolemia, shock, cardiac dysrhythmias, diaphragmatic hernia, abdominal trauma, fractures, or central nervous system injury. The animal must be stabilized by correcting life-threatening problems before anesthetizing the animal and attending to the wound.[17,20,23] The wound should be covered with a sterile dressing to prevent further contamination until definitive wound treatment can be performed.

SURGICAL TECHNIQUE

Assessment of the Wound

Once the animal has been stabilized, the surgeon can begin to care for the wound. Thorough evaluation of the body part must be done to determine nerve function, vascular integrity, and the extent of tissue damage.[17] Nerve function must be evaluated before the patient is sedated or anesthetized. The animal must be restrained and free of pain for adequate wound inspection and treatment.[3,14] General anesthesia is usually the best method of restraint for adequate wound care.[3,14] It has been said that the 11 most common sources for wound contamination are the surgeon's nasopharynx and 10 fingers; therefore, the surgeon should wear a cap, mask, and gloves while handling the wound.

One must protect the wound while preparing the surrounding skin. One of the most common methods of protecting the wound is to pack it with sterile gauze sponges moistened with saline.[14,17,33,34] Another acceptable method is to fill the wound with sterile, water-soluble jelly.[14,33,34] Once the surrounding skin has been prepared, this material is wiped or washed from the wound, along with any foreign material that has adhered to it.[33]

An ample area surrounding the wound is clipped free of hair with electric clippers. All loose hair should be vacuumed away. Hair at the wound edges can be trimmed with scissors dipped in mineral oil. This causes the hair to stick to the scissors instead of dropping into the wound. It is advisable to have a separate pair of clippers used only for preparing contaminated or infected wounds, as this may help to avoid contamination of other surgical sites.[33]

Once the skin surrounding the wound has been clipped free of hair, the gauze sponges are removed from the wound and replaced with fresh ones.[17,33] The skin is then surgically prepared making certain that the skin antiseptics do not enter the wound. Before preparing the area around wounds on the head, an eye ointment should be instilled to protect the cornea and conjunctiva.[33] Once the surrounding skin has been prepared, the gauze sponges are removed and the superficial wounds are cleaned with sterile saline. All visible foreign material must be removed.[14,33] The surgeon must avoid contaminating the surrounding skin with material removed from the wound.

Once the wound and surrounding skin have been prepared, the entire wound must be inspected to accurately assess the extent of the damage. The astute surgeon will recognize that the extent of skin trauma does not always correlate with the trauma to deeper tissues.[3,20] This is particularly true of puncture wounds and those caused by bite wounds. Once the extent of damage has been determined, the wound must be carefully debrided. All but the most simple lacerations should be debrided in the operating room.

Debridement

Debridement may be defined as the removal of devitalized tissue and foreign material from the wound.[17,22] It is the most important single factor in the management of contaminated wounds and is frequently neglected since the discovery of antibiotics.[15]

After the wound has been inspected and the extent of damage has been assessed, the animal is moved to the operating room, and the skin surrounding the wound is given a final scrub. Scrubbing, gowning, gloving, and draping procedures should follow the standard principles of aseptic surgery.

The goal of debridement is to convert a contaminated or infected wound into a surgically clean wound. It is difficult to standardize the methods of debridement, since the technique will vary depending on the type, location, and duration of the wound, and the manner in which the wound was sustained.[17,33,34] There are two basic techniques: *layered* and *en bloc* debridement. Layered debridement is most common and involves removing devitalized tissue and foreign material beginning at the skin and proceeding to the wound depths.[33,34]

Badly damaged skin lacking capillary bleeding should be removed initially, because of its tendency to suppurate and become infected.[15,33,34] Although skin is precious and essential to wound closure,[33,34] it is preferable to remove devitalized skin and graft the wound later, rather than to leave the necrotic skin.[15] Determining skin viability in a fresh wound is often difficult.[17] Viable skin should blanch under pressure, with a rapid return of color when the pressure is released, and should bleed when cut. If there is still doubt about skin viability, the area can be reinspected in 48 hours. Secondary excision can be performed if necessary.[33,34]

Wounds frequently have skin flaps that have been separated from the underlying tissue. Venous return is the critical factor in skin flap survival.[33,34] Skin flaps containing trapped blood appear turgid and hard, and restoration of venous drainage is the key to flap survival. Unduly pale or bruised skin should be excised from a flap. A skin flap that is a little dusky on one end, with no distinct demarcation between normal and abnormal skin, probably has adequate venous return. A dorsally based flap is more likely to survive than a ventrally based flap that is folded back on itself, kinking its blood supply.[33,34]

After the skin has been debrided, all deep tissue that is dead, has a poor blood supply, or is heavily contaminated should be removed if possible.[15] This is particularly true of subcutaneous fat and muscle.[15,20] Contaminated fat should be liberally excised back to a healthy plane that is free of blood stain.[34] Muscle that is friable or mushy, has dirt ground into it, does not bleed when cut, does not contract when stimulated, or is darker or paler than surrounding muscle should be considered nonviable.[17,33,34] Such muscle should be completely excised. Generally, large amounts of muscle are expendable, and it is better to remove muscle than to experience the consequences of liquefaction necrosis and possible clostridial infection.[34]

Blood vessels, nerves, and tendons may also be damaged, particularly in wounds involving the extremities. These structures should not be debrided with the same vigor as skin, muscle, and fat.[17,20,33] If nerves and tendons are encountered, they should not be sacrificed unless they are totally severed. Any frayed ends should be trimmed, but definitive repair should not be attempted at the time of initial debridement. Exposed tendons, nerves and blood vessels should be covered with tissue to prevent further damage.[17,20,33] Once the wound has healed, severed tendons or nerves can be repaired with a greater chance of success than if repair is attempted initially.[33] Lacerations in large vessels can be sutured; however, this is generally not necessary unless collateral circulation is impaired.[33] These vessels can usually be ligated, provided collateral vessels are intact.

En bloc debridement is used for wounds in areas where there is excess tissue. It is the most certain method of removing devitalized and contaminated tissue.[9,34] This form of debridement may have limited use in wounds of the extremities or in wounds with exposed blood vessels, nerves, or tendons.[9] It can be accomplished by packing the wound with sterile gauze and suturing the overlying skin to hold the gauze in place. The entire wound is treated as a tumor by excising the mass with the margin of normal tissue so the gauze in the wound is never exposed.[34]

Enzymatic debridement may provide an alternative to surgical debridement. Enzymatic debridement is indicated for severely injured animals that are poor anesthetic risks and for wounds in which surgical debridement could result in injury to healthy tissue.[33] In the latter circumstances, the enzyme "decides" what tissue will be removed and what tissue will remain, and the surgeon does not take the chance of removing questionable tissue that may revitalize and be useful in reconstruction.[33] Topical proteolytic enzymes have been shown to enhance the effectiveness of topical antibiotics through their fibrinolytic activity.[15] Even though topical proteolytic enzymes are fibrinolytic, their short-term use has been shown not to interfere with healing of experimental wounds.[26] The disadvantages of enzymatic debridement include the expense, the time required to remove dead tissue, and insufficient debriding action.[33] The author has also observed considerable discomfort in some animals that had wounds enzymatically debrided.

Lavage

Lavaging of wounds to remove bacteria and foreign material is essential to wound management, along with debridement.[3] Wound lavage is beneficial in removing foreign material and separated particles of tissue, and in removing, diluting, or decreasing the number of bacteria.[5,9,17,27,33,34] Sterile isotonic saline and lactated Ringer's solution are good wound irrigants. Simple, low pressure irrigation delivered by bulb syringe or gravity removes large contaminant particles and reduces the number of bacteria in the wound.[5,9,15,17,27,33,34] Increasing the volume of lavage solution decreases the incidence of infection.[15,33] However, studies have shown that continuous and pulsatile high-pressure (10–15 psi) lavage are much more effective in reducing wound contaminants and bacteria than conventional (bulb syringe) methods.[5,27] It has been shown that high-pressure lavage can also cause damage by injecting irrigant solutions into tissues adjacent to the wound. However, the excellent cleansing capacity of high-pressure lavage appears to outweigh this side effect, since heavily contaminated wounds that were subjected to this treatment healed primarily without infection.[37] It has been suggested that high-pressure lavage be reserved for heavily contaminated wounds.[9,10] A compromise for lavage of moderately contaminated wounds might be to deliver the irrigant solution with a 35 ml syringe and a 19-gauge needle. This system delivers the fluid to the wound at about 7 pounds per square inch of pressure.[33]

Topical Antimicrobials

Surgeons seem to possess an almost irresistible urge to instill antiseptics or antibiotics into open wounds. The most commonly used antiseptic in veterinary surgery is povidone-iodine solution. There is tremendous controversy over the effects of antiseptics on wound healing and on decreasing wound infection.[6,10,17,19,20,25,31,36] Two similar, yet independent, studies were done to determine the efficacy of 10 percent povidone-iodine in decreasing the incidence of surgical wound infections. In one study, there was a significant reduction in wound infections,[31] whereas there was no significant reduction in wound infection in the other.[6] In another study, there was a significantly increased infection rate in wounds irrigated with a 5 percent povidone-iodine solution and a significantly decreased infection rate in wounds irrigated with 1 percent povidone-iodine solution.[36]

Other antiseptic solutions include 2 percent chlorhexidine and benzalkonium chloride. In a recent study comparing antiseptics in dogs, little tissue reaction was seen with chlorhexidine and povidone-iodine in noninoculated wounds.[1] Excellent control of wound sepsis using 0.5 and 1 percent solutions of chlorhexidine, and a high concentratioin of benzalkonium chloride (1:2,500), was reported. Povidone-iodine solution was slightly less effective, even at the high concentrations (0.5 percent).[1]

Although topically applied antibiotics are advantageous, the surgeon should consider the potential cytotoxic effects of these drugs before they are used.[33] Topical antibiotics may be used in unstable animals that are unable to undergo surgical wound debridement, thereby decreasing the number and growth of wound bacteria until debridement can be performed.[33] Systemic antibiotics may not be effective in such animals because of poor blood supply in severely traumatized wounds. Topical antibiotics can be placed at the very site where they are needed and in concentrations that would be too toxic for systemic use.[33]

Commonly used antibiotics include neomycin, cephalothin, sodium ampicillin, and penicillin.[29] Since many wounds are contaminated with penicillin resistant strains of *Staphylococcus* sp., the use of penicillin or sodium ampicillin is probably not efficacious. The use of neomycin–bactracin–polymyxin has been shown to be effective against staphylococcal and streptococcal infections in minor skin trauma.[16] A mixture of 4 grams of cephalothin sodium or carbenicillin indanyl sodium per liter of saline has resulted in an excellent kill of staphylococcal and streptococcal organisms and good results against *E. coli*. Neomycin (10 grams per liter of saline) has given excellent results against these organisms and against *Klebsiella* and *Pseudomonas*.[11] A 0.25 percent neomycin/saline solution has been used by the author and is especially helpful in wounds contaminated with *Pseudomonas*.

Regardless of whether or not a surgeon chooses to use topical antibiotics or antiseptics in treating wounds, they should never be used in lieu of meticulous surgical debridement.

Systemic Antibiotics

The primary indication for systemic antibiotic therapy in treating traumatic wounds is to prevent septicemia that may be associated with wound infection. Systemic antibiotics may not reach adequate concentrations in the wound to be locally effective, especially in severely traumatized wounds that have a poor blood supply,[30,33] therefore, their value in preventing wound infection is questionable. Systemic antibiotics may be a valuable adjunct to initial wound management, but they should never be used as a substitute for good judgment and meticulous wound debridement.

Antibiotic prophylaxis refers to the administration of antibiotics to patients without evidence of established infection, with the objective of reducing subsequent septic complications.[21,24] When deciding whether to use prophylactic antibiotics, one must consider not only the wound, but the causes of wound contamination and the animal's ability to respond to the contamination. If bacterial contamination or tissue trauma is great enough to present a serious risk of infection, the surgeon should consider supplementing the animal's natural resistance with antibiotics.[24]

Although there are no rigid rules or formulas that will always give optimum results, there are guidelines that may assist the surgeon in determining the need and form of antibiotic use.[12,21,24,30,33]

1. The antibiotic should be present in the wound in effective concentrations before surgical debridement and be maintained only as long as the risk of new bacterial contamination exists.

2. Bacterial cultures should be taken, and the antibiotic used for prophylaxis should be effective against the organisms expected to be encountered.

3. Narrow-spectrum antibiotics should be used to minimize the risk of superinfection and the emergence of resistant pathogens. Broad-spectrum antibiotics needed to combat resistant infections should not be used for prophylaxis.

4. A bactericidal drug is preferred and should be given parenterally before debridement begins.

5. Antibiotic prophylaxis should be limited to some clean wounds, all clean contaminated wounds, and some contaminated wounds.

The most common error in using prophylactic antibiotics is continued administration beyond the necessary time period.[21]

The veterinary surgeon frequently treats wounds that are obviously infected at presentation. Therapeutic systemic antibiotics should be used according to the same guidelines followed for the use of prophylactic antibiotics, except that therapeutic antibiotics should be administered for at least 4 or 5 days after clinical signs of infection have subsided.[33] The antibiotic should not be changed unless the animal's condition worsens or culture and sensitivity results indicate otherwise. If septicemia develops, a blood culture should be obtained. If the organism recovered on culture is not sensitive to the antibiotic being used, an effective antibiotic should be substituted.[33]

Primary Versus Delayed or Secondary Closure

After wound debridement and lavage have been completed, the surgeon is faced with the decision of whether to close the wound primarily. This decision should be based on the amount of devitalized tissue and contamination that remains, the assessment of local tissue defenses, hemostasis, time lapse since injury, and the assurance of careful wound observation after closure.[33] Whether primary or delayed closure should be done after initial wound debridement is not always an easy decision. "When there is any dubiety, leave the wound open" is a good maxim to follow.[7]

Primary closure should be reserved for wounds that have little chance of infection and dehiscence after closure.[9,33] Since the danger of wound infection is greater in a closed wound than in an open wound, this method of closure should be performed under ideal conditions, and the surgeon should be convinced that healing will progress uninterrupted.[33] Most wounds that are caused by sharp objects (e.g., glass) usually contain little devitalized tissue and low levels of bacteria. Following meticulous debridement and lavage, these wounds usually heal without complication after primary closure.[33]

If management by delayed closure has been elected, the wound is not closed until local infection has been controlled, which is usually 3 to 5 days after wounding.[9,33] Delayed closure is beneficial because it provides the opportunity to examine the progression of healing, allows redebridement if necessary, and provides for wound drainage. Managing contaminated wounds by delayed closure also reduces the chance of infection.[9,33,35] The wound should be covered with a sterile dressing and kept under a pressure bandage, if possible. If further minimal debridement is expected, the author has found applying sterile gauze sponges directly to the wound to be helpful. Nonviable tissue that adheres to the sponge is removed during bandage changes. Some viable cells may also be removed using this technique, but the advantage of removing nonviable tissues outweights this disadvantage. If further debridement is not necessary, the wound should be covered with a sterile nonadherent dressing. This dressing should permit absorption of exudates from the wound. The bandage may initially need changing two to three times daily, depending on the quantity and quality of the exudate. As the amount of wound drainage decreases, the bandage may be changed less frequently. Aseptic technique should be followed during bandage changes, in order to avoid further wound contamination. Suture closure is performed when the tissues appear healthy and the exudate consists of small amounts of nonodorous, serous drainage.[9] Additional debridement may be necessary before wound closure.

Secondary closure usually implies the formation of granulation tissue and is performed later than 5 days after injury.[9,33] The skin edges become adherent to underlying tissue, once granulation tissue has formed. Apposition of the skin edges will be possible only after dissecting them free. The skin edges can be closed over the granulation tissue. Some surgeons prefer to excise the granulation tissue before closing the skin.[33]

Sutures and Wound Closure

·   Any foreign material left in a wound, including sutures, will increase the incidence of infection.[2,8,32,33] Ideally, sutures should be avoided in contaminated wounds, but this is not always practical. Therefore, the surgeon's choice of suture should be based on sound principles, including the chemical and physical properties of the suture. Regardless of the suture material used, certain principles should be followed. The suture should be of small diameter. Tying sutures tightly or incorporating large masses of tissue within sutures should be avoided. The surgeon should strive to bury the least amount of suture material possible. Knots should be precisely placed with no more throws than necessary for a secure knot.

Surgical gut is rapidly absorbed in infected wounds because of the presence of inflammatory cells and their associated proteolytic enzymes, which destroy the suture. Therefore, surgical gut should be used sparingly in contaminated or infected wounds.[33] The author limits the use of surgical gut in such wounds to ligation of blood vessels.

Polyglycolic acid and nylon sutures are frequently used in contaminated or infected wounds. These sutures are not affected by the products of inflammation, and their breakdown products may have some antibacterial properties.[8,33] The author prefers to use polydioxanone suture (PDS) because it is also not affected by inflammation and is a monofilament, absorbable suture. Additionally, it has good handling qualities and good knot security.

When closing a wound, the surgeon should strive to accurately appose tissue layers and eliminate dead space. Failure to eliminate dead space allows the accumulation of blood or serum within the wound. These fluids may effectively isolate bacteria from tissue defense mechanisms, thereby promoting infection. If dead space cannot be eliminated by sutures, placement of a drain may be necessary. Other indications for drains include wounds in which foreign material, contamination, or devitalized tissue remain in the deeper tissues. There are two general types of drains. Active drains employ the use of suction to actively remove tissue fluids and foreign material from the wounds. Passive drains work by capillary action and gravity flow, and should always be placed at the most dependent portion of the wound. Drains should be covered with a sterile dressing whenever possible. This allows assessment of the quality and quantity of drainage, minimizes the chance of ascending infection, and deters animals from chewing and possibly removing the drain.[33] The bandages should be changed as necessary, depending on the volume of drainage. Drains should be removed as soon as possible, generally when there is little or no drainage from the wound.

Hematomas adversely affect wound healing by providing a medium for bacterial growth and by isolating bacteria from tissue defenses. The surgeon should therefore strive for meticulous hemostasis before closing a wound. If hemostasis cannot be adequately achieved, then the surgeon should consider using drains, as discussed previously.

Wounds should be closed under minimal tension. If wounds are closed under excessive tension, dehiscence may result because of tissue strangulation or sutures tearing through the tissue. If wounds cannot be closed without excessive tension, they should be left open to heal by contraction and epithelization or covered with a skin flap or graft. Wounds should not be covered with skin flaps or free grafts until infection is controlled.

REFERENCES

1. Amber EI, Henderson RA, Swaim SF, Gray BW: A comparison of antimicrobial efficacy and tissue reaction of four antiseptics on canine wounds. Vet Surg 12:63, 1983
2. Bellenger CR: Sutures, part II. The use of sutures and alternative methods of closure. Comp Cont Ed 4:587, 1982
3. Bojrab MJ: Wound management. Mod Vet Pract 63:867, 1982
4. Bojrab MJ: Wound management. Mod Vet Pract 63:791, 1982
5. Brown LL, Shelton HT, Bornside GH, Cohn I, Jr.: Evaluation of wound irrigation by pulsatile jet and conventional methods. Ann Surg 187:170, 1978
6. deJong TE, Vierhout RJ, vanVroonhoven TJ: Povidone-iodine irrigation of the subcutaneous tissue to prevent surgical wound infections. Surg Gynecol Obstet 155:221, 1982
7. Dudley HAF: Wounds and their treatment. In Hamilton Bailey's Emergency Surgery. 10th Ed. John Wright & Sons Ltd, Bristol, 1977
8. Edlich RF, Panek PH, Rodeheaver GT et al: Physical and chemical configuration of sutures in the development of surgical infection. Ann Surg 177:679, 1973
9. Hackett RP: Delayed wound closure: a review and report of use of the technique on three equine limb wounds. Vet Surg 12:48, 1983

10. Hackett RP: Management of traumatic wounds. Proc Am Assoc Eq Pract, 363, 1978
11. Hoeprich PD: Chemoprophylaxis of infectious diseases. In Hoeprich PD (ed): Infectious Diseases—Modern Treatise of Infectious Processes, Harper & Row, Hagerstown, 1977
12. Holmberg DL: Prophylactic use of antibiotics in surgery. Vet Clin North Am 8:219, 1978
13. Hunt TK: Surgical wound infections: an overview. Am J Med 70:712, 1981
14. Jennings PB: Traumatic wounds. In Bojrab MJ (ed) Current Techniques in Small Animal Surgery. 2nd Ed. Lea & Febiger, Philadelphia, 1983
15. Jones RC, Shires GT: Principles in the management of wounds. In Schwartz SI (ed) Principles of Surgery. 3rd Ed. McGraw-Hill, New York, 1979
16. Leyden JJ, Sulzberger MB: Topical antibiotics and minor skin trauma. Am Fam Physician 23:813, 1981
17. Lipowitz AJ: Management of gunshot wounds of the soft tissues and extremities. J Am Anim Hosp Assoc 12:813, 1976
18. Meakins JL: Pathophysiologic determinants and prediction of sepsis. Surg Clin North Am 56:847, 1976
19. Mulliken JB, Healey WA, Glowacki J: Povidone-iodine and tensile strength of wounds in rats. J Trauma 20:323, 1980
20. Neal TM, Key JC: Principles of treatment of dog bite wounds. J Am Anim Hosp Assoc 12:657, 1976
21. Nichols RL: Use of prophylactic antibiotics in surgical practice. Am J Med 70:686, 1981
22. Peacock EE, VanWinkle W: Repair of skin wounds. In Wound Repair, 2nd Ed. WB Saunders, Philadelphia, 1976
23. Perry MO: Metabolic response to trauma. In Schwartz SI (ed): Principles of Surgery. 3rd Ed. McGraw-Hill, New York, 1979
24. Riviere JE, McCall-Kaufman G, Bright RM: Prophylactic use of systemic antimicrobial drugs in surgery. Comp Cont Ed 3:345, 1981
25. Rodeheaver G, Bellamy W, Kody M et al: Bactericidal activity and toxicity of iodine-containing solutions in wounds. Arch Surg 117:181, 1982
26. Rodeheaver G, Marsh D, Edgerton WT, Edlich RF: Proteolytic enzymes as adjuncts to antimicrobial prophylaxis of contaminated wounds. Am J Surg 129:537, 1975
27. Rodeheaver GT, Pettry D, Thacker JG et al: Wound cleansing by high-pressure irrigation. Surg Gynecol Obstet 141:357, 1975
28. Rodeheaver G, Wheeler CB, Rye DG et al: Side-effects of topical proteolytic enzyme treatment. Surg Gynecol Obstet 148:562, 1979
29. Scherr DD, Dodd TA: In vitro bacteriological evaluation of the effectiveness of antimicrobial irrigating solutions. J Bone Joint Surg 58-A:119, 1976
30. Schilling JA: Wound healing. Surg Clin North Am 56:859, 1976
31. Sindelar WF, Mason GR: Irrigation of subcutaneous tissue with providone-iodine solution for prevention of surgical wound infection. Surg Gynecol Obstet 148:227, 1979
32. Stashak TS, Yturraspe DJ: Considerations for selection of suture material. Vet Surg 7:48, 1978
33. Swaim SF: Management of contaminated and infected wounds. In Swaim SF (ed): Surgery of Traumatized Skin: Management and Reconstruction in the Dog and Cat, WB Saunders, Philadelphia, 1980
34. Swaim SF: Trauma to the skin and subcutaneous tissues of dogs and cats. Vet Clin North Am 10:599, 1980

35. Verrier ED, Bossart KJ, Heer FW: Reduction of infection rates in abdominal incisions by delayed wound closure techniques. Am J Surg 138:22, 1979
36. Viljanto J: Disinfection of surgical wounds without inhibition of normal wound healing. Arch Surg 115:253, 1980
37. Wheeler CB, Rodeheaver GT, Thacker JG et al: Side effects of high-pressure irrigation. Surg Gynecol Obstet 143:775, 1976

6 | Trauma of the Respiratory Tract

Daniel C. Richardson

The respiratory systems of the dog and cat consist of the lungs and the upper and lower air passageways that lead to the sites of gaseous exchange. The thoracic cavity is also a part of this system and plays an important role in ventilation by expanding and constricting to enhance air movement. It also protects the lower respiratory tract from the effects of trauma. An intact diaphragm enhances the movement of air into the lungs.

The purpose of the respiratory system is to deliver oxygen to the blood while removing carbon dioxide in exchange. This gaseous exchange is critical in maintaining cellular metabolism and organ function. Disruption of respiration due to trauma involving one or more portions of the respiratory system may lead to hypoxia, hypercarbia, and eventual death.

Trauma is one of the leading causes of respiratory system failure in a companion animal practice. Pathology of the respiratory system can result from motorized vehicles, falls from buildings, penetrating wounds from bullets or arrows, and violent encounters with other animals.

A recent study of dogs and cats suffering limb fracture(s) from motor vehicle accidents demonstrated a significant association with thoracic trauma. The incidence of thoracic injury in dogs with forelimb fractures was 34 percent versus 33 percent of those with hindlimb fracture. In cats this was found to be a 22 percent incidence with forelimb fracture and 13 percent with hindlimb fracture. Thus, trauma to the rear of an animal does not preclude the need to evaluate thoroughly for thoracic injury.[38]

The respiratory tract begins at the nares. Air that is inspired into the nasal cavity is warmed and humidified. It is directed to the pharynx, an area common to the digestive as well as the respiratory tract. The adjacent larynx allows careful regulation of the amount of air entering or leaving the lungs. This is a musculocartilagenous structure that also aids in vocalization. The glottis is an opening in the larynx, the diameter of which is controlled by abductor and adductor muscles within the larynx. Abduction on inspiration allows air to enter the trachea; adduction occurs during swallowing or gagging to prevent aspiration. The trachea's primary function is to provide a conduit for the passage of air to the lung proper. Cilia trap foreign matter to prevent its entrance into the lungs. The mainstem bronchi are similar in structure and function to the trachea. The bronchi enter the lung as branching bronchioles which become alveolar ducts that connect to alveolar sacs. These sacs are comprised of alveoli where gaseous exchange occurs between inspired air and the blood.

In order for ventilation to occur, the lungs must expand, drawing air in, and collapse, expelling "waste" gases. This is accomplished through an interaction of mechanisms and inherent tissue properties. The lungs are elastic in nature, expanding and collapsing readily. This expansion and collapse occurs simultaneously with movement of the chest wall, made up of ribs, intercostal muscles, and the diaphragm. The thoracic cavity is lined with pleura that reflects onto the lungs. This pleural reflection forms two symmetrical halves, separated by the mediastinal space. If the mediastinum is complete, as in man, atmospheric air entering one half will not cause the opposite lung to collapse.

Controversy exists as to the complete or incomplete nature of the mediastinum in the dog and cat. Clinical cases and a series of experimental animals have been documented that have acute or chronic pathologic processes involving only one pleural cavity.[42] Pneumomediastinum can also exist without a corresponding pneumothorax. These are important considerations when attempting therapy. If unilateral disease exists, then drainage techniques and local antibiotic instillation must be directed to the affected area. However, the mediastinum is quite friable, and bilateral disease may eventually develop from disease that was once limited to a hemithorax. Unilateral pleurocutaneous defects and tension pneumothorax often result in bilateral lung collapse.

A pleural space is naturally formed between the parietal and visceral layers. A thin, noncompressible, nonexpansible layer of fluid occupies this space. This fluid acts much like a thin layer of water between sheets of glass, holding them together, yet allowing them to slide with minimal friction. In this manner, the lung is held to the internal thoracic wall. The lung tries to "pull away" as the intercostal muscles expand the chest, creating the subatmospheric pressure necessary for the inward movement of air into the alveolar space. As the chest contracts, again through actions of the intercostal muscles, the inherent elasticity allows the lungs to collapse and expel a portion of the gases within the lung. The alveoli avoid collapse due to a layer of surfactant maintaining the surface tension. Ventilation also depends greatly on the diaphragm, since it accounts for the major changes in intrathoracic volume.

Disruption of the respiratory apparatus can occur anywhere along the respiratory tract. In the dog and cat, rarely is a single element involved. Generally, multiple areas and organ systems are affected. Trauma to the upper airway (nares to thoracic inlet) is generally evident on initial examination and primarily involves mechanical disruption of airflow. Fractures involving the nares and

mandible rarely interfere with respiration. However, swelling in the orophar-
yngeal region, blood aspirated through the glottis, and neurologic disruption
can result in decreased airflow for proper ventilation. A tracheotomy may be
indicated in order to fulfill the first goal of cardiopulmonary resuscitation, maintenance of a patent airway. Crushing injuries or laceration of the cervical trachea are relatively uncommon, but when they do occur, they are most often
related to bite wounds. If the tracheal integrity is disrupted, subcutaneous
emphysema is usually present.[24,25,27,29,39]

Damage to the thorax and its contents is the most frequently encountered
respiratory tract trauma. The thorax is relatively resistant to the effects of
trauma; thus, injuries resulting in damage to its contents are of a violent nature.
The ribs provide excellent protection, due to their flexible nature. The very
nature of the lungs, being elastic and air-filled, aids in their protection as well
as helping to protect other vulnerable thoracic contents.

Decreased ventilation due to trauma can occur in many ways. The gaseous
exchange can be disrupted at the alveolar level due to fluid (edema, blood)
accumulating within the alveoli. A solid mass, air, or fluid within the pleural
space will displace the lung, decreasing its overall capacity. Disruption of the
diaphragm can result in decreased intrathoracic volume. If abdominal organs
translocate into the pleural space through a tear in the diaphragm, overall lung
volume can be greatly compromised. Fractured ribs may result in lacerations
of the lung parenchyma, decreased ventilatory movement due to pain, or actual
loss of the "bellows" activity in the case of a flail segment. Pleurocutaneous
defects can result in complete collapse of the lungs as atmospheric air enters
the thorax, breaking down the pleural interface between the lung and throacic
wall.

Disease states induced by trauma can affect (1) primary conducting airways, (2) chest wall, (3) pleural space, and (4) lungs. Each area is discussed
in this chapter, as it relates to respiratory tract trauma. Therapeutic considerations are aimed specifically at the respiratory tract, but when managing the
traumatized patient, one should not fail to consider other body systems, as
well, in the definitive management.[1,23,29]

PRIMARY CONDUCTING AIRWAYS

The pathway from the environment to the lungs is bridged by the upper
airway. It consists primarily of the nares, nasal cavity, oropharynx, and tracheobronchial tree. Injuries to this region are generally obstructive in nature,
causing a decrease in inspired gases.

Nares/Nasal Cavity

Trauma to the nasal cavity resulting in fractures of the facial bones and
turbinates can occlude the nasal passages due to swelling and/or hemorrhage.
Since dogs and cats breathe primarily through the nose, dyspnea and open

mouth breathing is usually quite evident. Most animals will survive nasal obstruction. The more immediate life-threatening concern is to evaluate the patient for a patent airway distal to the nasal cavity. Aspiration of blood can lead to various degrees of obstruction to smaller airways.

Mouth breathing, when there is nasal obstruction, is the animal's way of reducing upper airway resistance. Air flow resistance is normally lower in the oropharynx when compared to the nasal cavity. Thus, open mouth breathing should markedly lower ventilatory efforts. While mouth breathing reduces airway resistance, ventilatory efforts and subsequent energy expenditures may actually increase. It becomes very important to reduce stress in the patient by minimizing handling and increasing inspired oxygen concentrations to assist respiration. Inspired oxygen can be increased via facemask, oxygen chamber, transtracheal catheter, or tracheal intubation if necessary.

Continued mouth breathing results in ventilation with air from the environment, without the benefit of the humidification and warming that the nasal tissues provide. The turbinate structures act as an air conditioner, warming and humidifying inspired air and extracting heat and water from the expired air.[11] This countercurrent exchange process functions as an auxiliary thermoregulatory mechanism and protects the respiratory tract from harsh, sudden changes in inspired air. Continuous mouth breathing can result in drying of the respiratory tract epithelium. This drying results in a less efficient function of the lower airway.

Hemorrhage from nasal trauma is generally controlled by keeping the patient quiet and avoiding the use of drugs that suppress the gag reflex, thereby decreasing the chances of aspiration. Continued bleeding requires further action. Inadequate clotting factors can be temporarily improved by fresh whole blood transfusions. In the event of normal clotting parameters but continued bleeding, topical agents such as epinephrine or thrombin, diluted in sterile water or sterile isotonic saline, may be used. Direct spray application or packing of the nasal cavity with epinephrine or thrombin-soaked gauze can be attempted. These methods usually require some sedation or possibly general anesthesia. If a specific, large vessel (e.g., sphenopalatine or infraorbital artery) can be located as the bleeding source, ligation is the preferred treatment. A final resort in continued, uncontrollable hemorrhage in the dog, is to ligate the carotid arteries in the midcervical region. This will reduce blood flow to the nares and potentially allow hemostasis. Packing of the nasal cavity is generally done in conjunction with the ligation.

Fractures involving the nasal cavity rarely require surgical correction. Palpation and visual inspection are generally adequate to determine clinical significance of nasal cavity fractures. However, further radiographic evaluation is indicated if large areas of bony defects or instability are noted. Free bone fragments within the nasal cavity may form sequestra with subsequent osteomyelitis and nasal drainage. Once the patient is stabilized, these are removed via nasal exploratory surgery. Defects in the bone overlying soft tissues may result in a nonhealing wound. This is particularly the case with oronasal defects resulting in oronasal fistulas. Fractures to the maxilla and hard palate resulting in large areas of instability can be stabilized with interfragmentary wire fixation and pins. Oral bracing techniques may also be considered. Small fragments may be removed and discarded. Most defects that result will eventually be bridged with soft tissue, including periosteum, and later with bone.

Oropharynx

The oropharynx is common to the digestive and respiratory tracts. The larynx, framed by the cricoid and thyroid cartilages and containing the paired arytenoid cartilages and the epiglottis, surrounds the entrance to the trachea. Its main function is to maintain an open airway during respiration and to close the airway during deglutition. This function is maintained through a close interaction of laryngeal muscles and nerves.

Impairment of laryngeal air flow due to trauma is rare. However, when dysfunction of the larynx occurs, it can be immediately life-threatening. Direct trauma from dog bites or other penetrating wounds may disrupt the larynx from its hyoid attachments or allow the encroachment of soft tissue into the airway. Cervical trauma may injure the vagus and/or recurrent laryngeal nerves, resulting in paresis or paralysis of the intrinsic laryngeal musculature.

Direct trauma rarely requires surgical intervention. Severe swelling and soft tissue damage may require anti-inflammatory drug therapy and a tracheotomy. Associated dysphagia may necessitate a feeding tube such as pharyngostomy or tube gastrostomy.

If laryngeal muscle dysfunction is present, a tracheotomy may be necessary to maintain air passage until function returns. When irreversible damage to the nerve supply has been determined, more definitive surgical therapy may be necessary. A partial arytenoidectomy, arytenoid lateralization, ventriculocordectomy, or tracheostomy may be indicated.[19]

Tracheobronchial Tree

Trauma to this portion of the respiratory tract sufficient to produce rupture is relatively uncommon. Penetrating wounds from animal bites and gunshot injuries usually predominate. Blunt trauma can occasionally disrupt the tracheobronchial tree. Regardless of the etiology, a cardinal sign related to tracheobronchial tree injury is subcutaneous emphysema.[39]

Puncture wounds or lacerations to the trachea may result in localized subcutaneous emphysema. Locating the lesion may require bronchoscopy. Severity is judged clinically by evaluating the chronicity of the emphysema. Static conditions probably indicate a self-sealing wound. Large wounds of the ventral trachea take on the function of a crude tracheostomy.

Tracheal disruption resulting from nonpenetrating trauma generally occurs within 2.5 cm of the corina[7] and can result in pneumothorax, pneumomediastinum, subcutaneous emphysema in the cervical and thoracic inlet region, and hemoptysis. Disruption occurs experimentally when a sudden and severe pressure is applied over a large area of the chest wall while the back remains fixed in position. A sudden compression of the ventrodorsal diameter with lateral widening of the chest results. Distraction in the cranial region ruptures the trachea. Incidence of rupture increases when the lungs are inflated and the glottis is closed.[7]

Rupture within the mediastinum can result in pneumomediastinum alone. Diagnosis requires radiographic evaluation. However, most cases of pneumomediastinum have concurrent subcutaneous emphysema in the cervical region. This can spread with time to involve the entire body, due to air spreading along the fascial planes to the loose subcutaneous tissues. A traumatized patient with a puffy, crackling, crepitating subcutaneous emphysema can be a dramatic presentation. Distress may be present due to local pressure on the trachea, but rarely is the trapped air life-threatening. However, continued build-up of pressure within the mediastinum and subsequent rupture into the pleural space may result in a rapid, life-threatening pneumothorax.

An obvious palpable defect in the trachea may aid in diagnosis and subsequent plans for repair. However, continued buildup of subcutaneous air and/or increased respiratory distress may indicate the need to assess the tracheal integrity via bronchoscopy. The lesion can be identified and definitive repair planned.

Repair of tracheobronchial lesions ranges from observation and cage rest to resection of the involved area and reanastomosis. Patients with cervical subcutaneous emphysema that is not ongoing in nature will respond to conservative management. Close observation for worsening signs and medication to reduce excitement and coughing are indicated. If the defect is on the ventral surface of the cervical trachea and open to the environment, management much like a tracheotomy site is sufficient. These will eventually granulate, seal, and epithelialize if kept clean. Extensive lacerations to or complete severance of the tracheobronchial tree requires more aggressive surgical efforts.

Tracheal defects may be closed primarily, undergo delayed closure, or be allowed to granulate. Primary closure can be utilized with laceration-type wounds as well as with total severance of the trachea. Lacerations may be closed by simple interrupted monofilament, nonabsorbable sutures placed in adjacent tracheal cartilages. Some wound debridement may be necessary if tissue viability is questioned. Complete separation of the tracheal rings may occur from a penetrating wound or as a result of a "whiplash" injury. The latter generally occurs in the cranial mediastinum and is best approached via a right cranial thoracotomy.[30] Three to four sutures should be placed 2–3 rings away from the primary line of closure to relieve tension at the anastomotic site. Closing is then completed with interrupted sutures of monofilament nonabsorbable material apposing adjacent cartilage rings and the dorsal ligaments. Markedly contaminated wounds may require a temporary tracheostomy distal to the injury to allow open treatment of the associated tissue injuries. This can be followed by definitive repair in a few days. Surgical repair must achieve good apposition of the tracheal mucosa without tension, in order to decrease the chance of dehiscence or stricture.[22] The tracheal mucosa has very poor abilities to fill in gaps and the trachea is relatively intolerant to tension at the anastomotic site. Up to one-third of the canine trachea can be removed with successful reanastomosis.[7]

The use of bandages to combat subcutaneous emphysema secondary to tracheal disruption should be avoided. If the trapped air does not increase in volume, it will resolve on its own with time. If the spread continues, surgical repair is indicated. Bandages redistribute the trapped air to other areas of the body, at best. The real danger may arise if a tear in the cervical trachea continues to leak, increasing pressure under the wrap, and subsequently collapsing the trachea. The attempt to treat the underlying cause should be the primary goal of therapy for subcutaneous emphysema.

CHEST WALL

The chest wall is comprised of the ribs and intercostal muscles. The chest wall along with the diaphragm makes up the boundaries of the thoracic cavity. This space is of primary importance to ventilation and circulation. The chest wall performs both a protective and a mechanical function for the thoracic organs. Damage to the chest wall may occur from penetrating or nonpenetrating wounds. Injury will result in a change in the expansibility of the lungs and thorax. This expansibility is termed *compliance* and is recorded as the volume increase in the lungs for each unit increase in intra-alveolar pressure.

Rib Fractures

Fractured ribs may be single or multiple. They generally occur in older animals as the bone becomes less malleable.

Simple fractures with minimal displacement may cause little more than a slight decrease in ventilatory movement due to pain. Slightly more serious in nature is the underlying trauma to the lung tissue resulting in hypoxemia. This is often seen in association with rib fractures and will be discussed under lung contusions. If trauma is sufficient, fractured ribs can displace and lacerate the underlying lung parenchyma as well as abdominal organs such as the liver and spleen.

The flail chest has long been represented as one of the more serious chest wall injuries. This condition results when two or more adjacent ribs are fractured proximally and distally. The resulting free floating segment moves paradoxically with ventilatory movements. A similar condition arises in very young animals with only proximal rib fractures due to the flexibility of the distal rib cartilage.

Although the respiratory function is altered by the paradoxical movement of the chest wall, the primary impairment is due to the underlying lung damage. Without concurrent pathology of the underlying lung, the paradoxical movement of a flail segment does not usually result in hypoxemia.[16] The most important lesion associated with a flail chest is pulmonary contusion. It has been stated that this is probably the primary cause of respiratory complications in these patients.[6,41]

The physiological changes that occur with flail chest injuries include decreased vital capacity, reduced functional and residual capacity, loss of compliance and an increase in airway resistance.[31] The mechanical effects, underlying lung contusion and the pain associated with rib fractures, cause the patient to expend a great deal of effort to expand the lungs. Treatment of patients with rib fractures or a flail segment should be directed toward the relief of pain, minimizing mechanical disruption of the chest wall, and, most importantly, reversing the underlying pulmonary pathology.

Treatment is dependent on the severity of the rib fracture. Single, non-displaced fractures rarely require more than conservative management. Observation for complications may be all that is needed. Displaced fragments may require some sort of internal stabilization to avoid laceration of the underlying lung parenchyma. Several techniques using wire and pins have been advocated.[28] On rare occasions, laceration of intercostal vessels may result in excessive hemorrhage. Surgical evaluation and ligation may be indicated. Severe pain and resultant hypoventilation may require the use of a local intercostal nerve block[27] or systemic analgesics.

Flail segments have been stabilized with external coaptation. The coaptation device can fix the flail segment either medially in a collapsed state or laterally in an expanded state. The advantage to an expanded fixation is that the ribs are more likely to heal in a normal anatomic alignment. Various techniques have been described.[6,9,25,27] These include stabilizing the flail segment to adjacent ribs or to an external splint. This maintains the segment in alignment with the normal chest wall. Open surgical reduction and stabilization can also be used, especially in cases of associated severe soft tissue damage requiring reconstruction and closure.

Chest wall trauma involving comminuted rib fractures and large soft tissue defects may require a major reconstruction effort. Techniques have been described utilizing marlex mesh, plastic spinal plates, omentum, and diaphragm advancement.[9,12,13,18] Intercostal muscle tears may be seen, especially as sequelae to a bite wound. Lung tissue can herniate through the defect, resulting in an impaired ventilation. These defects, when occurring as a single entity, can be repaired in a manner similar to routine thoracotomy closure.[28]

PLEURAL SPACE

Pneumothorax

Pneumothorax is the abnormal accumulation of air within the pleural space, and is one of the most common sequela to thoracic trauma.[27] Pneumothorax may be classified as simple open or tension. In either case, lung collapse occurs due to the accumulation of air between the parietal and visceral pleura. The lung volume decreases, resulting in a decreased ventilatory capacity. The bellow action of the chest wall is eventually diminished. Additionally, the small airways may fill with fluid or hemorrhage as a result of the trauma. This further reduces the ventilation/exchange abilities of the lung. The end result is severe hypoxemia.

Various causes of pneumothorax have been documented. Penetrating wounds and lung lacerations from fractured ribs have been mentioned previously. Pneumothorax can also arise from nonpenetrating blunt trauma and has been seen to spontaneously occur, usually secondary to some underlying lung pathology.[43]

Simple Pneumothorax (Closed Pneumothorax)

This is a condition generally associated with blunt, nonpenetrating thoracic trauma. Air leaks into the pleural cavity through a wound in the lung. Diagnosis is initially based on physical findings of increased rate and depth of respiration, hyperresonance of this chest wall and radiographic evaluation.

Management of pneumothorax is based on the severity of clinical signs and the initial response to therapy. If the animal is in respiratory distress, thoracocentesis is indicated. However, if the patient is tolerating the pneumothorax and is stable, the stress of excessive handling should be avoided. The animal should be allowed to rest quietly but be under frequent observation. If the animal's cardiopulmonary status remains stable for 24 hours post-trauma, and follow-up radiographs indicate no further increase in air accumulation, the pneumothorax will probably undergo eventual resolution. Most parenchymal injuries with a subsequent air leak are self-limiting.

Open Pneumothorax

In open pneumothorax the pleural cavity is exposed to the atmosphere through an open wound in the chest wall. A relatively small lesion, in comparison to the diameter of the glottis, may allow adequate ventilation. Air entering the pleural cavity on inspiration can be expelled on expiration. Large wounds, however, result in severe hypoventilation. More air is drawn through the chest wall defect than can be pulled into the lung fields via the glottis.

Treatment requires immediate coverage of the wound. An airtight seal is best accomplished with the placement of gauge impregnated with ointment over the wound. However, emergency management may be adequate with a cloth or the palm of the hand. Aspiration of the pleural cavity is performed if respiratory distress is evident. Definitive therapy involves soft tissue would management, subsequent closure, and chest drainage. Thoracocentesis alone may be adequate. However, underlying parenchymal injury may necessitate a tube thoracostomy to maintain negative pressure while the air leak seals spontaneously. If the lung leak continues after closure of the pleurocutaneous defect, a tension pneumothorax may result.

Tension Pneumothorax (Pressure Pneumothorax)

Tension pneumothorax results from a closed pneumothorax and a lung leak that does not seal. A similar condition results with an open pneumothorax in which the soft tissues surrounding the opening into the pleural cavity act as a one-way valve. This results in air entering the pleural space and becoming entrapped. The lungs progressively compress, and intrathoracic pressures eventually become great enough to impair venous return to the heart. The tolerance level of pneumothorax in the dog is quite high. Intrapleural volumes of air equalling 3.5 times the functional residual capacity are tolerated. However, this condition can rapidly result in hypoventilation and circulatory collapse. The thorax is maximally distended, while ventilatory movements are greatly reduced. If percussed, the thorax is usually hyperresonant. The impending circulatory collapse is evaluated through the weak, rapid peripheral pulses. As the intrapleural pressure approaches atmospheric pressure, respiratory embarrassment progressively increases.

Diagnosis can be confirmed by thoracocentesis, with subsequent relief of distress. Radiography may not be possible until repeated aspirations allow a return to a less compromised state. If the aspiration of the air from the pleural space does not resolve the pneumothorax, a tube thoracostomy is indicated. This may be unsuccessful if the leak persists or is excessively large. In these instances, bilateral tube thoracostomy may be indicated. Thoracotomy and definitive repair of the injury may be indicated if air continues to be withdrawn in the chest tube for 48–72 hours without any sign of resolution.

Hemothorax

Blood accumulating in the pleural space is a common sequela to thoracic trauma. The clinical severity of hemothorax is dependent upon the amount of blood present, the source of the bleeding, and associated injuries. Bleeding may arise from the pulmonary vessels, a relatively low pressure system, or be associated with systemic vasculature arising from the chest wall, heart, or diaphragm.

Parenchymal and small vessel tears generally are self-limiting when normal clotting mechanisms are intact. Clotting is assisted by a tamponade effect created by the blood accumulating within a fixed space. Free air from concomitant pneumothorax can also contribute to this tamponade effect. This effect places pressure on a low pressure leak and enhances hemostasis. Oftentimes, this amount of hemorrhage goes unrecognized clinically. The concurrent pneumothorax is usually of greater concern to the patient's respiratory function.

Bleeding from the chest wall, diaphragm or primary cardiac vessels routinely continues despite build-up of intrapleural blood. These higher pressure vessels overcome any tamponade effect. Clinical signs are dependent upon the amount of hemorrhage and the acute nature of the blood loss.

Local impairment of respiration is associated with the space-occupying effect of the blood. Lung expansion is compromised. Atelectasis and right-to-left shunting occur, as they do in pneumothorax. The end result is a decreased ventilation–perfusion ratio. Clinically significant signs are dyspnea, restlessness, decreased heart and lung sounds, cyanotic mucous membranes, and a decreased resonance on thoracic percussion.

Systemic signs accompanying the respiratory distress are related to the amount of blood loss. Large volumes of blood escaping into the thoracic cavity may result in signs consistent with hypovolemic shock.

Diagnosis is based upon clinical signs and radiography, and is confirmed with thoracocoentesis. These cases are similar to those presenting with pneumothorax, and in actuality, most have some degree of pneumothorax. Those animals demonstrating no obvious source of bleeding, yet with a history of trauma and signs of hypovolcmic shock, merit a high index of suspicion for bleeding of thoracic origin. Radiographs demonstrate a fluid density between the parietal and visceral pleura. Thoracocentesis is necessary to confirm the presence of hemothorax.

Free blood in the thorax is thought to clot, then undergo rapid defibrination.[29] This results in radiographic signs of fluid indistinguishable from any other liquid substance within the thorax. However, with the history of recent trauma, fluid densities generally represent blood until proven otherwise. Due to minimal potential for contamination, this blood is usually quite acceptable for autotransfusion (see Chap. 2). Many of the blood clotting factors are unavailable but the blood is an excellent source for volume reexpansion. Free blood in the thorax does not indicate an absolute need to perform thoracocentesis. Only in the face of a local space-occupying effect on the lungs does it need to be removed immediately. Systemic hypovolemia from hemothorax is best treated by fluid volume expansion with crystalloids initially, followed by a blood transfusion if indicated.

The bleeding may be self-limiting. Serial radiographs are indicated to evaluate progression or cessation of hemorrhage. Radiographic evidence of continued hemorrhage along with deteriorating clinical signs may require surgical exploration and ligation of any bleeding vessels. Intercostal vessels may be easily located near fractured ribs where they can be ligated without entering the thorax. Bleeding from the major thoracic vessels may require a thoracotomy. A median sternotomy is indicated if the exact location of hemorrhage is unknown. This allows the majority of the thoracic cavity to be explored. Angiography may be helpful prior to surgery to pinpoint the source of bleeding. The patient's condition will dictate the decision to perform this diagnostic procedure. Following a thoracotomy, postoperative thoracic drainage is indicated. The chest tube is removed when hemorrhage has ceased, packed cell volume is stabilized, and negative pressure is reestablished.

Chylothorax

Chyle is the milky fluid taken up by the lacteals from intestinal content during digestion. It is composed of lymph and triglyceride fat droplets (chylomicrons) in a stable emulsion. Chylothorax comes from a mixture of intestinal and thoracic lymph and can result from any episode of thoracic trauma that disrupts the thoracic duct. The thoracic duct originates in the abdomen at the cisterna chyli and passes cranially on the right side of the diaphragm in association with the aorta. It passes almost the entire length of the mediastinum prior to emptying into the major veins.[33] The thoracic duct of the cat passes along the left side of the mediastinum. Thus, disruption of the thoracic duct or one of its collateral branches may occur in association with rib fractures, pneumothorax, hemothorax, diagphragmatic hernia, or pulmonary contusion. However, traumatic rupture is rare.[33]

Clinical signs are associated with decreased lung expansion from the space-occupying effect of the accumulating chyle. The signs are often slow (days to weeks) in onset. This can be due to an initial collection of chyle in the mediastinum prior to escape into the pleural space.[37] Another reason for this latent effect may be associated with the fact that the thoracic duct/lymph system is a low-pressure, relatively low-volume system, and thus the chyle is slow to accumulate.

Clinical and radiographic signs are similar to hemothorax patients. The primary difference is the lack of signs compatible with systemic blood loss. The onset of signs are rarely as acute as in hemothorax. Diagnosis is based on thoracocentesis and assessment of the fluid. The fluid is usually an opalescent milky color, and odorless on gross examination. Staining with Suden III allows light microscope visualization of chylomicrons. Solubility of the opalescence is demonstrated by the addition of ether to the fluid.

To distinguish between chylous and nonchylous effusions, triglyceride levels can be determined. In man, values greater than 110 mg/dl are highly suggestive of chylous fluid. If the values are equivocal, that is, between 50 and 100 mg/dl, then lipoprotein electrophoresis of the chyle as a final step is necessary to confirm the diagnosis.

Rare cases of pseudochylous (chyloid) effusions have been reported.[37] This effusion contains a high concentration of cholesterol cyrstals, probably as a result of degenerative pleural endothelial processes.[37] Chylomicron globules are usually not seen when examined microscopically.

Infection secondary to chylothorax is rare, due to the lecithin components of chyle that exhibit a bacteriostatic effect. However, thoracocentesis attempts and the inherent inflammatory response to chyle result in pleural adhesions.[37]

Treatment generally involves thoracic drainage of the accumulated chyle, utilizing single or multiple thoracocentesis. This allows re-expansion of the lungs, and in some cases the duct lesion heals spontaneously. Persistent cases may require chest drains for 7 to 10 days to allow the lungs to remain expanded and the duct to heal. Conservative management is often unsuccessful, thereby resulting in the need for surgical intervention with duct ligation.[5] Surgical ligation is sometimes followed by the formation of another form of pleural effusion that may continue for days to weeks. Pleurodesis combined with underwater continuous pleural drainage is sometimes necessary to eventually achieve resolution of the pleural effusion.

Diaphragmatic Hernia

Diaphragmatic hernias may be congenital or acquired. The vast majority are acquired and are the result of a forceful trauma to the abdomen.[41] A traumatic blow to the abdomen results in increased intra-abdominal pressure. The diaphragm, being the most flexible boundary of the abdomen, balloons into the thoracic cavity. If the glottis is open, the lungs deflate, and no counter pressure is applied to the cranially advancing diaphragm. The result is a large pleuroperitoneal pressure gradient, and the diaphragm tears.[41] Pneumothorax is an uncommon accompanying event. Penetrating injuries may also result in a loss of diaphragm integrity.

The diaphragm is necessary for normal respiration, yet the defect in the diaphragm is seldom life-threatening. Adequate compensation by other abdominal and thoracic muscles occurs. This is evidenced by accentuated movement of the abdomen and thorax during ventilation. Rib fractures and underlying pulmonary pathology (contusion, edema) are more contributory to the dyspnea seen in the early stages of this disease.

If the rent is of sufficient size, abdominal viscera (primarily liver, intestine, stomach, and/or omentum) readily enters the pleural space. This results in a space-occupying lesion and partial collapse of the lungs. The atelectatic lung fields are poorly ventilated but continue to be perfused. This results in an abnormal ventilation–perfusion ratio, and the animal becomes hypoxic. Venous return and cardiac output can be markedly altered by reduction of negative pressure within the thorax and local compression from the herniated viscera. Hypoventilation can result in hypercapnia and a respiratory acidosis.

If the viscera move freely back and forth from thorax to abdomen, ventilatory changes may be transitory. However, strangulation or adhesion of an abdominal organ within the thorax can create a progressively deteriorating condition. A gas-filled bowel loop may become strangulated, resulting in signs compatible with bowel obstruction and endotoxemia due to ischemia and bowel wall necrosis. The stomach may lodge within the thorax and become dilated if the pyloric and cardiac regions are occluded by kinking or torsion. This condition may be rapidly fatal. The liver may be associated with hemothorax if it has been severely traumatized and its bleeding surface enters the thorax. More commonly, the liver becomes partially incarcerated in the defect. This can result in a hydrothorax, as transudation of fluids occurs from the serosal surface. If constriction occurs as the defect attempts to heal, this transudation is enhanced. Pleural effusion (hydrothorax) is a result of disturbance to normal dynamic equilibrium between systemic vascular hydrostatic pressure, plasma colloid osmotic pressure, and negative intrapleural pressure.[30] These disturbances can occur with diaphragmatic hernias and subsequent abdominal viscera herniation into the thoracic cavity.[27]

Clinical signs are quite variable in relation to a diaphragmatic hernia. They may be intermittent, constant, acute, chronic, life-threatening, or debilitating. In general, the signs relate to mechanical compression of the lungs and thoracic vessels and/or obstruction of the gastrointestinal tract.

Diagnosis is based on a history of abdominal trauma, clinical signs related to the thorax and abdomen, physical exam findings, and radiography. The majority of cases, whether acute or chronic, allow some degree of preparation for surgery. Surgery as an emergency procedure is indicated only when the animal seems in imminent danger of death, such as in a dilating stomach trapped within the thorax, a strangulated loop of bowel, or deteriorating signs in spite of medical therapy.

Surgical repair is necessary for a definitive cure of a diaphragmatic hernia. A ventral midline incision extending from the xyphoid to the umbilicus is recommended. A median sternotomy may be necessary to reduce the herniated viscera and reconstruct the rent, especially in very chronic cases. Site predilection is primarily for the muscular portion of the diaphragm and quite often results in a separation from the costal attachments. Reconstruction can usually be attained with primary suturing. Continuous suture patterns are generally best to achieve quick closures and airtight seals. A simple continuous or Ford-Interlocking pattern is simple and effective. Absorbable versus nonabsorbable suture material is probably a minor consideration. Both are effective if used properly. Nonabsorbable, monofilament swaged-on suture is easy to handle, has adequate strength in the proper sizes, and will maintain strength, especially in cases of marked tension and constant motion. Despite the suture pattern and material, care must be taken to avoid iatrogenic damage to the lungs, vessels, and nerves passing near and through the diaphragm. All cases are best managed with the intraoperative placement of a thoracic chest tube to allow reestablishment of negative pressure and short-term monitoring for continued collection of air or fluid. The tube is usually removed within 24–48 hours.

Large defects may be seen in cases that are long-standing as a result of tissue contracture and in penetrating wounds that destroy a large segment of diaphragm. These may require more innovative closure methods. Many materials and tissues have been advocated to close these large defects. Synthetic mesh such as polypropylene (Marlex), dacron (Mersilene), and silastic sheets have been used. Organs such as the stomach, spleen, colon, and renal fascia have been utilized to "plug" the hole.[40] Omentum has also shown promise as a biologically compatible structure to fill the defect.[14]

LUNGS

Pulmonary Contusion

Pulmonary contusion is a bruising of the lung, manifested by the presence of edematous fluid and blood withing the air spaces (alveoli) and interstitial areas of the lung parenchyma.[28] Most victims of blunt thoracic trauma suffer some degree of pulmonary contusion.[25] Upon impact, thoracic wall compression results in a tearing and crushing of lung tissue. With rapid dissipation of this force, the resultant negative pressure causes more damage. Hemorrhage from torn vessels fills and obstructs the alveoli and bronchioles. Bleeding and edema also occur within the interstitial spaces. Alveoli rupture and collapse, resulting in areas of atelectasis. Perfusion to the alveoli continues but ventilation is interrupted. This results in a venous admixture and subsequent hypoxemia.[24] Traumatic lung cysts have been incriminated with severe pulmonary contusion and parenchymal damage. The presence of these air-and/or fluid-filled cysts indicates severe thoracic trauma and the patient is at high risk for a pneumothorax.[2]

Clinical signs depend on the amount of lung tissue involved. Small, focal areas of contusion are not clinically evident in most cases. Greater area involvement results in tachypnea, varying degrees of respiratory distress, and, on occasion, hemoptysis. Auscultation may reveal harsh lung sounds. Occasionally, "quiet" areas are found with the stethoscope. If a very large area such as an entire lung lobe is involved, large areas may be ausculted where no air movement is occurring. Radiography is the definitive means of diagnosing this condition. The most severe physiologic manifestations of lung contusion are generally present within 2 hours of the injury.[31] Radiographic signs become evident within 6–8 hours. Clinical and radiographic resolution should begin within 24 to 48 hours post-trauma. Resolution is generally complete in 3 to 10 days.[28]

Treatment of contused lungs is based on the premise "do not harm." Most cases require little to no medical treatment and respond to conservative treatment consisting of rest and observation. Oxygen therapy, provided with an oxygen cage, face mask, or with nasotracheal or transtracheal methods will aid in combating hypoxia. Stressing the patient further by excessive restraint to keep a face mask in place should be avoided. The use of a transtracheal or nasotracheal catheter may be a less stressful way of maintaining an increased concentration of inspired oxygen. Antibiotics are indicated to cover secondary infections in the injured and devitalized lung parenchyma. Glucocorticoids are often indicated to reduce inflammation and concurrent pulmonary edema.

Fluid therapy must be used with caution. The anatomic and physiologic alterations caused by pulmonary contusion can be worsened with rapid administration of crystalloid solutions such as lactated Ringer's solution.[41] Shock therapy doses of 90 ml/kg may be indicated for improving the vascular volume but often result in a compromised pulmonary system due to the contribution to pulmonary edema. Fluid administration should always be accompanied by constant assessment of the animal's respiratory function. Increased moist lung sounds and dyspnea indicate a need for modification of fluid administration. Urine output at 2–3 ml/kg/hr is ideal for adequate kidney perfusion. Lack of urine production and continued fluid administration will result in a fluid overload, and the pulmonary system will be an early victim. Vascular endothelial damage and resultant fluid leakage will further compromise ventilatory ability. Use of colloid solutions, blood, or plasma may be a better approach if vascular expansion therapy is needed, as in the case of shock and contused lungs. Diuretics, bronchodilators, and tracheobronchial suction may be necessary in severe cases, in order to keep the airways open. Frequent positional changes, especially in recumbent patients, will help avoid hypostatic congestion and further atelectasis.

Pulmonary Edema

Pulmonary edema generally results as a primary event or a sequela to a disease process. It is defined as an abnormal accumulation of liquid and solute in the interstitial tissues, airways, and alveoli of the lung.[36] The two types of greatest concern in trauma are neurogenic pulmonary edema and shock lung syndrome.

Neurogenic pulmonary edema occurs following brain or head injury and is thought to be a result of increased intracranial pressure. This pressure stimulates liberation of catecholamines via a massive sympathetic discharge. Peripheral resistance increases with a concurrent rise in blood pressure increasing circulation to the pulmonary system. Resultant capillary damage allows fluid leakage over several days, even after pressures and flow return to normal. This fluid accumulation within the alveoli interferes with gas exchange. Respiratory compromise and possible suffocation can be the end result, if it is allowed to progress. Neurogenic pulmonary edema has also been a sequela to heat stroke, electrocution seizures, (following biting an electric cord) and hypoglycemia.[36] Therapy has been aimed at treating the inciting cause and attempting to reduce the alpha- and beta-adrenergic overactivity through the use of sympatholytic, antiepinephrine drugs, oxygen, and general anesthetic agents.[8,36]

Shock lung syndrome is an acute respiratory failure due to massive pulmonary edema. In man, it is also known as "adult respiratory distress syndrome." This disorder is due to increased pulmonary vascular resistance and altered pulmonary vascular permeability.[36] Various endogenous humoral agents and thromboemboli released following lung trauma are thought to combine with damaged pulmonary vascular endothelium. Therapy is symptomatic at best. Diuretics may assist in removing the edema fluid, and care must be taken to avoid exacerbating the edema by overzealous fluid administration.

DIAGNOSTIC/THERAPEUTIC TECHNIQUES

Transtracheal Catheter

Most thoracic trauma patients suffer from some degree of hypoxemia. Increased oxygen levels in the inspired air will greatly benefit patients with relatively normal alveolar perfusion but compromised ventilation. Oxygen masks are effective, but some animals may struggle excessively. An oxygen cage is not always available. A simple alternative for the delivery of oxygen to the lungs is a transtracheal catheter.

The technique of inserting a transtracheal catheter is similar to needle and catheter placement for a transtracheal wash. A large bore jugular catheter (14- to 16-gauge) is inserted into the trachea through the cricothyroid ligament, a palpable indentation adjacent to where the larynx joins the tracheal rings. The catheter is passed into the tracheal lumen. An intravenous drip set is modified to allow attachment of an oxygen source to the catheter. Nonhumidified oxygen will dry the tracheal mucosa if the oxygen is given over 4 to 5 hours. This procedure is generally temporary, until definitive therapy can be instituted.

Tracheotomy/Tracheostomy

Tracheotomy is an incision into the trachea. Tracheotomy is generally considered a short-term, emergency procedure, to bypass upper airway obstruction. Tracheostomy is the surgical creation of an opening into the trachea through the neck, with the tracheal mucosa brought into continuity with the skin.[4] This is a long-term or permanent procedure rarely performed for initial management of upper airway obstruction resulting from trauma.

Multiple techniques have been advocated for performing a tracheotomy. Two basic approaches allow ease of technique and efficacy. These include cutting transversely between two tracheal rings[19] or cutting longitudinally through 2 to 3 rings.[33] Creation of a window by removing a piece of tracheal cartilage increases the risk of stenosis at the tracheotomy site.

A simple ventral transverse incision between two rings approximately 4 or 5 tracheal rings below the cricoid cartilage allows the best placement of a tracheotomy tube. An endotracheal tube can be used in lieu of a tracheotomy tube.

A second technique involves a longitudinal incision through the ventral aspect of the trachea at the same level previously mentioned. The incision is only as long as needed to introduce an endotracheal or tracheotomy tube.

Management involves securing the tube in place by suturing it to the skin or tying it to the neck circumferentially with a piece of umbilical tape. The tube must be kept free of mucous and blood. Tracheostomy tube management requires constant monitoring of the patient. Periodic removal (at intervals of 30 minutes, initially), cleaning, and/or suctioning of the tube must be done routinely. A tracheostomy tube disrupts the normal ciliary action of the trachea as well as increasing mucous production due to mechanical irritation. There is a high risk of plugging with subsequent hypoxia that can be disastrous to the tracheotomized patient. When the tube is no longer needed, it is removed, and the tracheotomy site is kept clean and allowed to heal by second intention.

Permanent formation of a tracheostomy is rarely needed unless upper airway obstruction is permanent. If a tracheostomy is indicated, meticulous surgical technique, excellent client education, and careful postoperative management are essential.

The technique involves the creation of a window by excising 2 to 3 tracheal cartilages along their lateral and ventral surfaces. The trachea is moved toward the skin surface by bringing the sternohyoideus muscles together deep (dorsal) to the trachea. This reduces tension on the trachea/skin interface. The tracheal rings, ligamentous structures, and mucosa are then sutured to the skin edge.[20]

Postoperative management requires that the area be kept free of debris and mucous accumulation. It is also imperative that the animal not be allowed to swim, since aspiration of water would be likely.

Thoracentesis

The surgical puncture of the chest wall and entry into the pleural cavity for aspiration is termed *thoracentesis*. Other terms include *thoracocentesis* and *pleurocentesis*. This is usually the first step in establishing treatment for pneumothorax and diagnosis of fluid accumulations within the pleural space. It is also used to withdraw fluid from the pleural cavity to assist in radiographically identifying pleural masses or a diaphragmatic shadow.

Three basic techniques are readily available. The first and most common is the use of a large syringe, three-way stopcock, and hypodermic needle (18–20-gauge). The needle is inserted through the upper half of the 6th or 7th intercostal space. Care is taken to enter the pleural space by a gentle "pop" through the pleural lining. The needle should then be directed obliquely and ventrally, with the bevel directed toward the lungs, staying close to the ribs. This reduces the possibility of tearing lung tissue with the needle point. Avoid the intercostal vessels coursing posterior to each rib. A gentle negative pressure is maintained on the syringe as the needle is advanced.

A similar technique utilizes a bovine teat cannula. A local anesthetic may be required to allow a small skin incision and advancement of the cannula through the intercostal musculature. Due to its blunt tip, potential for iatrogenic lung trauma is reduced.

A third method utilizes an intravenous catheter. The sheath type of catheters (Venocath, Abbott Laboratories, North Chicago, IL 60064) work well for thoracocentesis. The technique is similar to simple syringe and needle aspiration. The only difference is that the needle stylet is retracted from the thoracic cavity after the catheter is introduced. This allows a relatively nontraumatic thoracocentesis, and the catheter can be safely advanced and withdrawn, increasing the likelihood of removing air or fluid. Generally, both sides of the thoracic cavity should be aspirated.

Tube Thoracostomy

A tube thoracostomy, or placement of a chest tube, is one of the most beneficial but often overlooked techniques in thoracic trauma. It is indicated when repeated thoracentesis is not effective and any time the thoracic cavity is opened to the atmosphere, then surgically closed. A chest tube allows continuous monitoring for air and fluid accumulation within the pleural cavity. The drain tube is also safer than repeated thoracentesis attempts.

Various thoracic drain tubes are available commercially. Generally, for the trauma patient, soft plastic or red rubber feeding or urinary catheters are quite effective. If the chest tube is to be maintained for more than a few hours, a regular thoracic drain tube should be used. The softer, less rigid urinary catheters may collapse or kink, thus reducing their efficacy.

A chest tube is best placed midthorax at approximately the 7th intercostal space. A local anesthetic is infused into the skin and subcutaneous tissues over the 7th to 10th intercostal spaces, with deep infusion of the muscles at the proposed site of tube penetration. A large curved hemostat is used to carry the drain through a subcutaneous tunnel and subsequently into the thoracic cavity. Bilateral placement may be necessary to adequately drain fluid and/or air from both sides of the chest. A clamp should be placed on the outside end of the tube to avoid introducing more air into the pleural space as the tube enters. Care should be taken to avoid the intercostal vessels posterior to the ribs. It is also critical that all fenestrations in the chest tube be placed within the thoracic cavity; holes under the skin or exposed to the atmosphere will worsen the pneumothorax. A pure-string suture is placed in the skin around the tube. Additional methods of suturing and taping can then be utilized to maintain the tube. Hemostats or other clamp devices must be maintained between aspirations. Otherwise, iatrogenic pneumothorax will result. Frequency of aspiration is dependent on the amount of air or fluid accumulating. Heimlich valves, one-way flutter valves, work well but may be less effective in smaller dogs and in cats. They can become clogged with blood, become dislodged, or simply give a false sense of security in a patient that should be monitored much more closely. Thus, frequent manual aspiration with secure air-tight clamping of the tube between episodes is strongly advocated.

Continued negative pressure or lack of fluid on aspiration probably indicates the need to remove the tube. The chest tube alone will cause pleural irritation and fluid production, thus the character (serous versus hemorrhagic) and amount should be the deciding factors. Radiographs of the thorax are indicated prior to chest tube removal. These films act as a baseline for future comparison and aid in determining if clinical signs, physical findings, and chest tube aspiration results all correlate. It is far better to leave a tube in place a little too long than to prematurely remove it, only to replace it when the animal begins to deteriorate. Various techniques are utilized to manage chest tubes in people. The use of water-sealed chest drains is very popular.[24] However, management of these devices in the dog or cat can be time consuming.

Removal of the chest tube should be done in one swift motion to avoid iatrogenic introduction of air into the pleural space. Pressure should be applied at the intercostal space where the tube entered the thorax. A light chest wrap with ointment impregnated gauze over the skin wound is indicated for 24 hours to avoid subcutaneous emphysema.

Thoracotomy

Thoracic trauma rarely requires a thoracotomy. However, when previously discussed techniques are unable to arrest the accumulation of air or fluid such as blood or chyle, open visualization of the thoracic cavity is indicated.

If a specific location of the injury is known, the best approach can then be chosen. Lateral thoracotomy may be performed on either side at any level, depending on the location of the lesion.[32] A median sternotomy[10,15,43] allows the majority of the thoracic cavity to be explored and is the better technique when exploring a chest for unexplained hemorrhage or air leaks. This technique is more time-consuming and technically more difficult than a lateral thoracotomy, yet it allows a rapid assessment of more structures within the thorax than do most other forms of thoracotomy.

Fortunately, very few thoracic trauma cases require a thoracotomy. Thoracentesis, oxygen therapy, tube thoracostomy, and enforced cage rest is sufficient in most cases.

SUMMARY

Trauma to the respiratory tract of the dog and cat is a common occurrence. Accurate assessment and management is critical to a successful outcome. The degree of trauma ranges from a barely perceptibly compromised respiratory system to life-threatening conditions of absolute and complete respiratory failure.

Rarely is respiratory trauma a single entity. Multiple body systems are involved. However, management of respiratory system injuries is often the most immediate link to success or failure in these polytraumatized cases.

Respiratory tract trauma management requires careful deliberation. Initial aggressive efforts to diagnose and stabilize the patient must be weighed carefully against the need to avoid excessive added stress to a patient who is barely maintaining adequate oxygenation.

REFERENCES

1. Aron DN, Emergency management of the muculoskeletal trauma patient. Comp Cont Ed 3:220, 1982
2. Aron DN, Kornegay, JN: The clinical significance of traumatic lung cysts and associated pulmonary abnormalities in the dog. Am Anim Hosp Assoc 19:903, 1983
3. Aronsohn M: Diaphragmatic advancement for defects of the caudal thoracic wall in the dog. Vet Surg 1:26, 1984
4. Berg P: Pneumothorax. p. 243. In Kirk RW (ed): Current Veterinary Therapy V. WB Saunders, Philadelphia, 1974
5. Birchard SJ, Cantwell HD, Bright RM: Lymphangiography and ligation of the canine thoracic duct: a study in normal dogs and three dogs with chylothorax. Am Anim Hosp Assoc 18:769, 1982
6. Bjorling DE: Flail chest: review, clinical experiences and new method of stabilization. J Am Anim Hosp Assoc 18:269, 1982
7. Bojrab MJ, Renegar WR: The trachea. p. 359. In Bojrab MJ (ed): Pathophysiology in Small Animal Surgery. Lea and Febiger, Philadelphia, 1981
8. Bradley RL, Keating ML: Neurogenic pulmonary edema in a cat. Feline Pract 9:26, 1979

9. Brasmer TH: The thoracic wall. p. 198. In Bojrab MJ (ed): Current Techniques in Small Animal Surgery I. Lea and Febiger, Philadelphia, 1975

10. Bright RM: Median sternotomy in the dog. Canine Pract 6:36, 1979

11. Bright RM: Nasal foreign bodies, tumors, and rhinitis/sinusitis. p. 335. In Bojrab MJ (ed): Pathophysiology in Small Animal Surgery. Lea and Febiger, Philadelphia, 1981

12. Bright RM: Reconstruction of thoracic wall defects using marlex mesh. J Am Anim Hosp Assoc 17:415, 1981

13. Bright RM et al: Repair of the thoracic wall defects in the dog with an omental pedicle flap. J Am Anim Hosp Assoc 18:277, 1982

14. Bright RM, Thacker HL: The formation of an omental pedicle flap and its experimental use in the repair of a diaphragmatic rent in the dog. Am Anim Hosp Assoc 18:283, 1982

15. Bright RM: Clinical and radiographic evaluation of a median sternotomy technique in the dog. Vet Surg 1:13, 1983

16. Cullen P, Modell JH, Kirby RR et al: Treatment of flail chest. Arch Surg 110:1099, 1975

17. Ellison GW, Trotter GW, Lumb WV: Reconstructive thoracoplasty using spinal fixation plates and polypropylene mesh. J Am Anim Hosp Assoc 17:613, 1981

18. Harvey CE: The larynx. p. 350. In Bojrab MJ (ed): Pathophysiology in Small Animal Surgery. Lea and Febiger, Philadelphia, 1981

19. Harvey CE, Goldschmidt MH: Healing following short duration transverse incision tracheotomy in the dog. Vet Surg 11:77, 1982

20. Hedlund CS et al: A procedure for permanent tracheostomy and its effects on tracheal mucosa. Vet Surg 11:13, 1982

21. Hedlung CS, Tangner CH: Tracheal surgery in the dog—Part II. Comp Cont Ed 9:738, 1983

22. Hunt CA: Chest trauma—the approach to the patient with chest injuries. Comp Cont Ed 7:527, 1979

23. Hunt CA: Chest trauma—specific injuries. Comp Cont Ed 8:624, 1979

24. Kagan KG: Thoracic trauma. p. 641. In Crane, SW (ed): Vet Clin North Am, Vol. 3. WB Saunders Co., Philadelphia, 3:641, 1980

25. Kagan KG: Results and complications of treatment of chylous pleural effusions in dogs and cats. Am Coll Vet Surg Abstracts 1984, Vet Surg 13 (1):53, 1984

26. Kolata RJ: Management of thoracic trauma. p. 103. In Wingfield WE (ed): Vet Clin North Am Vol. 1. WB Saunders, Philadelphia, 1981

27. Krahwinkel DJ: Lower respiratory tract trauma. p. 278. In Kirk RW (ed): Current Veterinary Therapy VI. WB Saunders, Philadelphia, 1977

28. Krahwinkel DJ: The trauma patient—diagnosis and therapy. Seminar, Univ of Tennessee, College of Veterinary Medicine, 1979

29. Krahwinkel DJ: Thoracic trauma. p. 268. In Kirk RW (ed): Current Veterinary Therapy VII. WB Saunders, Philadelphia, 1980

30. Mosely RV, Vernick JJ, Boty DB: Response to blunt chest injury: a new experimental model. J Trauma 10:673, 1970

31. Nelson AW: Thoracotomy. p. 275. In Bojrab MJ (ed): Current Techniques in Small Animal Surgery. Lea and Febiger, Philadelphia, 1983

32. Quick CB: Chylothorax: a review. J Am Anim Hosp Assoc 16:23, 1980

33. Rawlings CA: Tracheotomy. p. 69. In Wingfield WE, Rawlings CA (eds): Small Animal Surgery: An Atlas of Operative Techniques. WB Saunders, Philadelphia, 1979

34. Roudebush P, Burns J: Pleural effusion as a sequela to traumatic diaphragmatic hernias: a review of four cases. J Am Anim Hosp Assoc 15:699, 1979

35. Staats BA, Ellefson RD, Budahn LL et al: The lipoprotein profile of chylous and nonchylous pleural effusions. Mayo Clin Proc 55:700, 1980

36. Suter PF, Ettinger SJ: Pulmonary edema. p. 747. In Ettinger SJ (ed): Textbook of Veterinary Internal Medicine. 2nd Ed. WB Saunders, Philadelphia, 1983

37. Suter PF, Zinkl JG: Mediastinal, pleural, and extrapleural thoracic diseases. p. 840. In Ettinger SJ (ed.): Textbook of Veterinary Internal Medicine. 2nd Ed. WB Saunders, Philadelphia, 1983

38. Tamas P, Paddleford RR, Krahwinkel DJ: Incidence of thoracic trauma in conjunction with limb fractures following motor vehicle injuries in dogs and cats. Presented at the American College of Veterinary Anesthesiologists, Scientific Meeting, Atlanta, Oct. 6–7, 1983

39. Ticer JW, Brown GS: Thoracic trauma. p. 629. In Ettinger SJ (ed): Textbook of Veterinary Internal Medicine. WB Saunders, Philadelphia, 1975

40. Touloukian RJ: A "new" diaphragm following prosthetic repair of experimental hemidiaphragmatic defects in the pup. Ann Surg 1:47, 1978

41. Trinkle JK et al: Management of flail chest without mechanical ventilation. Ann Thorac Surg 19:4, 1975

42. von Recum AF The mediastinum and hemothorax, pyothorax, and pneumothorax in the dog. J Am Vet Med Assoc 171:531, 1977

43. Yohioka MM: Management of spontaneous pneumothorax in twelve dogs. Am Anim Hosp Assoc 18:57, 1982

7 | Abdominal Trauma

Stephen J. Birchard
Roger B. Fingland

Trauma to the abdomen is a well-recognized injury in veterinary medicine. Patients sustaining abdominal trauma present a diagnostic and therapeutic challenge, especially if multiple regions of the body are injured. In a study of 600 cases of motor vehicle accidents in dogs and cats, 36 percent had multiple region injuries while 70 percent had concomitant abdominal trauma and skeletal injury.[13] The establishment of priorities for victims of polytrauma is imperative. Intra-abdominal injuries such as a ruptured bladder are less obvious than skeletal injuries, yet are more life-threatening. A systematic and logical approach to trauma victims should result in early diagnosis and treatment of life-threatening problems.

The purpose of this chapter is to review the pathophysiology, diagnosis, and treatment of abdominal trauma. The decision of when to perform a laparotomy on a traumatized animal is given special attention.

MECHANISM OF INJURY

The type of trauma to the abdomen determines, to some extent, which organs are injured and the type of injury sustained. Blunt trauma usually causes injury to the liver and spleen, whereas penetrating trauma usually causes injury to the liver and intestine.[6] Recognition of the mechanism of injury may help the clinician to predict which organs have been damaged.

Blunt Abdominal Trauma

Encounters with motor vehicles, kicks, and falls commonly cause blunt abdominal trauma in dogs and cats. This type of trauma results in contusion, laceration, avulsion, or rupture of abdominal organs.[11] Intra-abdominal injury may not be immediately obvious after blunt trauma. Therefore, an aggressive diagnostic plan must be implemented to determine if laparotomy is necessary.

Damage to the abdominal wall may occur with blunt abdominal trauma. Severe muscle contusion or tearing can occur with minimal signs of external injury. Abdominal hernias may be seen in the inguinal, prepubic, flank, or other regions. Thorough palpation of the patient is necessary to detect these injuries.

Penetrating Trauma

Penetrating injuries to the abdomen cause perforation or laceration of the body wall and may involve abdominal organs. Stab wounds, gunshot wounds, and bite wounds account for the majority of these injuries. In general, the higher the velocity of the penetrating object, the more damage it causes.

Stab wounds or penetrating foreign bodies can lacerate tissue but usually create little contusion of the surrounding tissue. Even stab wounds that penetrate the abdominal cavity may *not* be associated with organ damage. In humans, one-third of abdominal stab wounds do not penetrate the abdomen, and of those that do penetrate, only one-half require laparotomy.[10]

Low-velocity gunshot wounds (e.g., .22, .38 caliber) create an area of tissue damage two to three times the diameter of the bullet.[1] Jacketed missiles do not deform, therefore creating less damage than missiles that do deform.

High-velocity gunshot wounds cause tremendous tissue destruction. Tissue damage can extend radially to 20–30 times the diameter of the missle due to concussion waves created by the bullet.[1] This destruction may not be obvious upon initial presentation. Aggressive surgical therapy is required for these patients. If these wounds penetrate the abdominal cavity, organ damage is likely and laparotomy is necessary.

DIAGNOSIS

The diagnosis of abdominal trauma may not be obvious because external injuries are not always present. This is particularly true in the case of blunt trauma.

The veterinarian's first priority is to treat life-threatening problems, such as shock, dyspnea, and hemorrhage. The second priority is to thoroughly examine the patient. One of the most important aspects of this evaluation is to determine if an exploratory laparotomy is necessary. The evaluation should begin with a complete history and physical examination followed by appropriate radiographic studies. Abdominocentesis or diagnostic peritoneal lavage may be used to further define the problem. Hematologic and biochemical parameters are also important in diagnosing problems related to abdominal trauma.

History

The clinician should obtain a history that is complete but does not delay treatment of the patient.

The physical examination and initial supportive measures should be done while the history is being obtained. The history may be misleading because the owner is often upset and not thinking logically. Simple questions that are pertinent to the animal's current problem should be asked, such as: what happened and how long ago, did you see the injury, has there been any bleeding and from what site, can the animal walk, have you see the animal urinate or defecate since the accident?[3] If the animal was injured with a weapon, the type of weapon used, the caliber of gun, and the distance from which it was used should be ascertained. The owners should also be asked about the animal's previous medical problems and current medications.

Physical Examination

The initial physical examination of the trauma patient should be a quick but comprehensive exam of all body systems. The cardiovascular and respiratory systems must be immediately evaluated for life-threatening problems. This section will deal primarily with the examination of the abdomen.

The first part of abdominal examination is external inspection. The hair is widely clipped over suspicious areas to evaluate for bruising, lacerations, hernias with or without evisceration, and entrance and exit wounds if penetrating trauma is suspected. The chest wall should also be carefully examined. Trauma to the caudal one-third of the chest is likely to result in hepatic or splenic injury. Extensive bruising in the inguinal area should raise the index of suspicion of urinary bladder or urethral rupture.

Bite wounds are always more severe than they appear externally. Small skin wounds are invariably associated with extensive damage to underlying muscle and fascia. These wounds should be probed with a sterile instrument to determine the extent of injury. Once the animal is stable, extensive wound debridement, irrigation, and drain placement are often necessary.

Gentle but thorough palpation of the abdomen should then be performed. Since hemoperitoneum is one of the most common consequences of trauma,[11] ballottement of the abdomen for fluid is recommended. Abdominal hernias, organ displacement, intra-abdominal or retroperitoneal masses, and pain may be evident on palpation. Lifting the animal by its front legs facilitates palpation of cranial abdominal structures.

Auscultation of the abdomen for intestinal sounds should be performed, but the results may be misleading. Bowel sounds were absent in only 64 percent of abdominal trauma patients who had positive diagnostic peritoneal lavages in one study.[18] Persistent absence of intestinal sounds is a more reliable sign of intra-abdominal injury.

Although the physical examination is a very useful tool in the diagnosis of abdominal injury, other tests frequently are necessary to confirm the presence or absence of organ damage.

Radiology

Abdominal radiographs should be obtained whenever abdominal trauma is suspected. This diagnostic step should not interfere with lifesaving therapeutic measures. It is important to obtain the radiographs before abdominocentesis or diagnostic peritoneal lavage are performed, since both techniques may cause iatrogenic pneumoperitoneum and/or hydroperitoneum.

Hydroperitoneum, evidenced radiographically by loss of detail and inability to define serosal borders, suggests the presence of blood, urine, bile, gastrointestinal fluid, transudate, or exudate from peritonitis. Abdominocentesis will help differentiate these fluid types. Free gas in the peritoneal cavity is suggestive of rupture of a hollow viscus, and emergency laparotomy is indicated.[19] Inability to outline the bladder on plain radiographs, coupled with hydroperitoneum, is suggestive of a ruptured bladder, and a positive contrast cystogram and urethrogram are indicated. Upper or lower gastrointestinal contrast studies may be necessary to rule out intestinal injury. If gastrointestinal perforation is suspected, aqueous iodine contrast agents have been recommended instead of barium to avoid the peritonitis associated with free barium in the abdomen.[5]

The retroperitoneal space should be carefully examined on abdominal radiography, when trauma is suspected. Inability to see the renal margins, and haziness or increased density caudal to the kidneys suggests retroperitoneal fluid. The fluid is either urine from a ruptured ureter or renal pelvis or blood from renal hemorrhage or vascular injury. An intravenous pyelogram should be performed whenever there is retroperitoneal fluid.

The integrity of the abdominal wall should also be examined on the plain radiographs. Abdominal hernias frequently can be seen radiographically. Bone structures should be carefully inspected for fractures or luxations.

It is important to remember that some radiographic changes associated with abdominal trauma may not be evident on the initial films. For example, focal peritonitis due to an intestinal perforation may take 3 days to show radiographic signs.[5] Repeat radiographic studies of the abdomen should be obtained if the animal's condition is deteriorating.

Abdominocentesis

Needle paracentesis of the abdominal cavity is a useful diagnostic technique. The skin should be aseptically prepared, and a four quadrant tap performed. Ideally, the patient should be standing. An 18- or 20-gauge needle (1–1½ inches long) is placed, and fluid is allowed to flow freely from the needle hub. Gentle abdominal massage sometimes facilitates the flow of fluid through the needle. Samples of fluid are saved for analysis (e.g., packed cell volume, total protein, cytology, chemistries). A free flow of nonclotted blood, urine, bile, or ingesta is a positive result.

Abdominocentesis is quick, inexpensive, and less invasive than peritoneal lavage. However, there is a high percentage of false-negatives.[7] Therefore, a negative finding does not rule out intra-abdominal injury.

Diagnostic Peritoneal Lavage

Diagnostic peritoneal lavage (DPL) is an accurate method for the diagnosis of intra-abdominal injury.[7,12] Although slightly more invasive and time-consuming than simple abdominocentesis, the results are more reliable.[12]

The technique begins with aseptic preparation of an area of skin around the umbilicus. A local anesthestic is injected subcutaneously 1 cm caudal to the umbilicus. A small (0.5 cm) incision is made in the skin and subcutaneous tissue, and then in the linea alba. A peritoneal dialysis catheter with stylet (Trocath) is placed through the incision. The stylet is removed, and the catheter is directed caudoventrally. Aspiration through the catheter is attempted first. If a positive aspirate is obtained (e.g., several ml of blood or urine), then lavage is unnecessary. If no fluid is obtained, 10–20 ml/Kg of lactated Ringer's solution is infused into the peritoneal cavity through the catheter. The patient is gently rolled from side to side, and the fluid is then siphoned from the abdomen. Samples of the fluid are saved for analysis. The catheter is withdrawn, and a suture is placed in the incision, if necessary.

The fluid is analyzed for packed cell volume, white blood cell count, cytology, amylase, bile, urea, and creatinine. Positive results are listed in Table 7-1.

Diagnostic peritoneal lavage allows early detection of significant organ damage before delayed signs occur (as with chemical peritonitis). The technique is reported to be approximately 90 percent accurate, and is more reliable than physical examination and abdominocentesis.[2,7,12] Reportedly, DPL allows detection of as little as 0.2 ml/kg of abdominal fluid.[12] Unnecessary celiotomies may be avoided by using DPL on more abdominal trauma cases.

Table 7-1. Interpretation of Peritoneal Lavage Fluid

Any of the following indicate intra-abdominal injury:
  1. Dialysis catheter fills easily with blood
  2. Grossly dark bloody or opaque lavage fluid
  3. More than 500 WBC/mm^3
  4. More than 200 IU amylase activity
  5. Presence of bilirubin
  6. Creatinine greater than serum concentration
  7. Bacteria
  8. Vegetable fibers
  9. Packed cell volume of lavage fluid greater than 5 percent
  10. Toxic neutrophils

Bjorling DE et al. Penetrating abdominal wounds in dogs and cats.
J Am Anim Hosp Assoc 18: 742, 1982, with permission.

Diagnostic peritoneal lavage has little value in the diagnosis of retroperitoneal injuries or diaphragmatic hernia. The radiographic signs and a thorough clinical evaluation must be relied upon for these injuries.

CBC/Serum Chemistries

When dealing with a trauma patient, there is not always time to obtain blood and urine for analysis. However, if emergency surgery is not indicated and the patient is stable, blood and urine analysis may prove helpful in injuries that are not immediately obvious.

Leakage of various body fluids into the abdomen produce changes in serum chemistries. Leakage of urine into the abdomen causes a marked increase in BUN. The serum creatinine may initially be normal, since it is a larger molecule than urea and is absorbed more slowly from the peritoneal cavity. Serum potassium is elevated with urine leakage into the abdomen. Bile leakage will cause increased serum bilirubin and icterus. Trauma to the pancreas results in elevations in serum amylase and lipase.

Elevations in creatine phosphokinase, SGPT, and SGOT are of questionable significance. These enzymes are frequently elevated even with mild trauma to the abdomen.

Peritonitis results in neutrophilia, frequently associated with a left shift. Stress alone can cause leucocytosis, so additional evidence of peritonitis should be present to confirm the diagnosis.

The packed cell volume and red blood cell count are not reliable tests for acute blood loss. Several hours are required for the PCV to drop after acute hemorrhage, and the pretrauma PCV is rarely known. Therefore, if intra-abdominal hemorrhage is suspected, serial PCVs (e.g., every 4–6 hours) should be obtained to establish a trend.

Local Exploration

Penetrating injuries caused by bullets frequently involve intra-abdominal injury. However, other forms of sharp trauma, such as bite wounds, do not always penetrate the abdominal cavity. Local exploration of the wound can be used to determine whether penetration of the peritoneal cavity has occurred. A local anesthetic (Lidocaine) may be used in conjunction with a narcotic (e.g., oxymorphone), if necessary, for sedation and analgesia. If the deepest recesses of the wound are found and abdominal penetration has not occurred, immediate laparotomy may not be necessary. However, if other evidence of intraabdominal injury is present, laparotomy should still be performed. If local exploration of the wound reveals penetration of the peritoneal cavity, exploratory laparotomy should be performed to determine the extent of damage.

The major advantage of local wound exploration is to prevent unnecessary laparotomy. If significant abdominal organ injury is present, exploratory laparotomy should be performed, followed by debridement of superficial wounds.

Good clinical judgment and interpretation of the diagnostic tests listed previously are necessary in order to determine which course of action to take.

INITIAL TREATMENT

All trauma patients require an immediate assessment of cardiopulmonary function. Establishment of a patent airway and adequate ventilation must be the first priority. If the animal is in shock, treatment with fluids and corticosteroids is indicated. Whole blood should be given if massive hemorrhage has occurred. The thorax should be thoroughly examined for injury, followed by evaluation of the abdomen.

The patient must be closely monitored after initial resuscitative efforts. Frequent observations of respiratory and cardiac function are necessary. Initial patient stabilization is necessary before pursuing diagnostics such as radiographs or diagnostic peritoneal lavagae. The main purpose of the diagnostics should be to determine whether emergency surgery is necessary. It is important to evaluate the patient's initial response to treatment. Continued deterioration necessitates more aggressive action.

THE DECISION TO OPERATE

The most difficult decision in the management of the abdominal trauma patient is whether or not to perform an exploratory laparotomy. A negative laparotomy is disappointing. However, it is more disappointing to delay the operation, have the patient die, and find a correctable lesion on post-mortem examination. If an error in judgment is made, it is better to be too aggressive than not aggressive enough.

A scheme for the initial management of the abdominal trauma patient is presented in Fig. 7-1. It is extremely important to keep all findings in perspective. The presence of blood in the abdomen does not always indicate the need for surgery, especially if the patient's circulatory status improves with fluid replacement. Persistent hemorrhage and deterioration of the patient in spite of appropriate therapy are indications for prompt surgery.

In the patient with blunt abdominal trauma, laparotomy is necessary only if there is clear evidence of intraperitoneal damage, such as a positive diagnostic peritoneal lavage or persistent intra-abdominal hemorrhage. In many cases, laparotomy is not necessary after blunt trauma and the patient will recover with conservative measures. Therefore, it is acceptable for the surgeon to be selective in choosing the patients needing surgery after blunt trauma. In contrast, penetrating trauma to the abdomen almost always requires immediate laparotomy. Gunshot wounds to the abdomen have been associated with a high percentage (70 percent) of intra-abdominal injury.[14] Therefore, prompt laparotomy should be performed in these patients. However, stab wounds to the abdomen have a much lower percentage (30 percent) of injuries requiring lap-

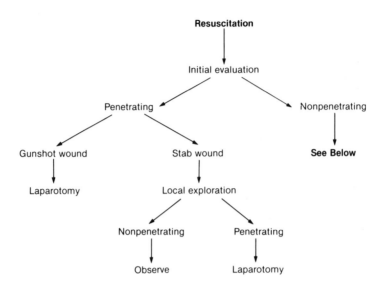

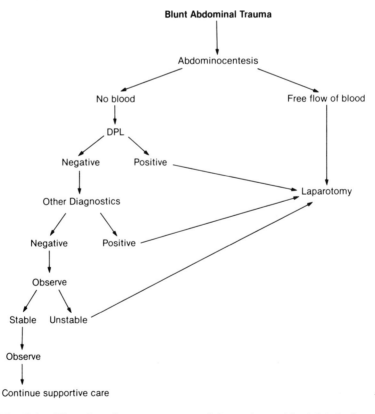

Fig. 7-1. Flowchart for management of the patient with abdominal trauma.

arotomy. Therefore, if clear evidence of organ damage is not seen after a stab wound or a bite wound, local exploration of the wound can be done to determine if abdominal penetration has occurred.[22] Laparotomy and a complete abdominal exploration should be done if penetration has occurred.

The value of diagnostic peritoneal lavage in making the decision to operate must be emphasized. Use of DPL has reduced the number of negative celiotomies to approximately 10 percent of those patients having blunt abdominal trauma.[8] It is a simple, practical technique that can be easily performed by the practitioner.

A negative celiotomy should not be considered a diagnostic failure. It is far better to perform a laparotomy and not find significant intra-abdominal injury than to procrastinate and have the patient die of a correctable lesion. Therefore, if any doubt exists, laparotomy should be performed.

The timing of surgery is another difficult decision. Will the patient benefit from initial conservative management? In most cases, yes. If the patient has had thoracic trauma in addition to abdominal trauma, and the thoracic problems are life-threatening, they must be treated before the laparotomy. If the patient is in shock from abdominal hemorrhage, fluids and corticosteroids must precede the laparotomy. Chemical peritonitis and uremia due to urine leakage into the peritoneum can initially be treated with abdominal drains. After 12–24 hours of drainage, along with fluid and antibiotic therapy, these patients are better candidates for the definitive surgical repair. Close observation of the patient during this preoperative period is critical. For example, the abdominal drain should be frequently checked for patency, and BUN, creatinine, and serum electrolytes should be measured to determine whether the patient is benefiting from the conservative approach. In the author's experience, the azotemia and hyperkalemia associated with uroperitoneum will markedly improve after placing abdominal drains and giving intravenous saline fluid therapy.

The abdominal exploratory operation should consist of a rapid but thorough examination of all organ systems. The first priority is to identify sources of hemorrhage (e.g., liver or spleen) and to control them. In the author's experience, if there has been major abdominal hemorrhage, opening of the peritoneal cavity may release the tamponade effect and allow additional bleeding. Hypotension results, necessitating rapid fluid administration.

The next priority is to control overt soilage of the abdomen, especially if leakage from the gastrointestinal tract is occurring. After repairing areas of gastric or intestinal rupture, lavage of the peritoneal cavity with copious amounts of warmed, sterile saline should be done. Systemic antibiotics should also be administered when contamination of the abdomen has occurred. The exploration can then be completed.

SPECIFIC INJURIES

Liver and Biliary System

The liver is the most frequently injured intra-abdominal organ in the dog.[13] Penetrating wounds often involve the liver, but more commonly the liver is lacerated or contused by blunt trauma. Frequently, multiple liver lobes are involved. Subcapsular hematomas can also occur secondary to trauma. These hematomas can develop into abscesses in 3–4 days if contaminated with bacteria, although this is a rare complication in the dog. Hemoperitoneum is the most common sign of liver trauma.

The management of liver trauma depends upon the type of injury. Shallow lacerations that are not bleeding require no treatment. Deep fractures should be debrided and closed with horizontal mattress sutures. Temporary occlusion (for up to 15 minutes) of the hepatic arteries can be used to control severe hemorrhage while repairing the wounds. The thumb and forefinger or umbilical tape through rubber tubing are used to occlude the arteries lying within the hepatoduodenal ligament. Large vessels in the hepatic parenchyma may require ligation. If the liver wound is too large to close, the greater omentum can be pedicled and used as a patch to fill the wound.[15] The liver wound and omentum are oversewn with a continuous suture. Lacerations at the periphery are best handled with partial lobectomy.

Trauma to the biliary tract can result in bile leakage and peritonitis. Gallbladder rupture or avulsion, or laceration of the hepatic, cystic, or common bile ducts can occur. Bile leakage into the abdomen may be overlooked if diagnostic peritoneal lavage is not performed. The presence of greenish black fluid or a positive Icto test on lavage fluid indicates bile in the peritoneal cavity. Icterus helps to substantiate the diagnosis. Severe peritonitis will result from bile leakage, but clinical symptoms may be delayed for several days.[20] If the peritonitis becomes septic, rapid deterioration of the patient's condition occurs.

A ruptured gallbaldder can be either repaired with sutures or simply removed (that is, a cholecystectomy can be performed). Duct avulsions or lacerations are repaired primarily, or stent tubing (e.g., a T-tube) is used to maintain patency of the duct while healing by second intention occurs. If the cystic duct alone is involved, cholecystectomy can be performed. Avulsion of the common duct from the duodenum may be managed with reimplantation, or an anastomosis between the gallbladder and duodenum (cholecystoduodenostomy).[6]

Spleen

Penetrating or blunt trauma can cause splenic injury. Hematomas, lacerations, or fragmentation of the splenic pulp can occur. Avulsion of splenic vessels results in profound bleeding. Splenic hematoma causes a splenic mass that may be visible radiographically. Large splenic hematomas should be removed surgically to avoid rupture and blood loss, even if several days have elapsed since the injury. Laceration of the splenic pulp or avulsion of splenic vessels causes hemoperitoneum, and laparotomy is sometimes required to control bleeding.

If most or all of the spleen is damaged, a total splenectomy should be performed. However, if 50 percent or less of the spleen is damaged, a partial splenectomy can be done.

Splenosis results from autotransplantation of splenic tissue to the omentum and other areas. It can occur after fragmentation of the spleen and appears as small red nodules in several locations in the abdomen.

Urinary System

The kidney is susceptible to contusion, hemorrhage, rupture, penetration, or avulsion of its vasculature. Injuries can occur with shearing forces across the renal parenchyma, or due a whiplash effect.[13] Renal hemorrhage fills the retroperitoneal space with blood. Rupture of the renal pelvis causes urine pooling in the retroperitoneal space. Intravenous pyelography (IVP) should be performed if retroperitoneal fluid is seen on plain films.

The tamponade effect of the retroperitoneal space may arrest hemorrhage, and laparotomy is not always required with renal injury. If the IVP does not demonstrate urine leakage, and the patient is stable, a conservative approach may be indicated. However, if bleeding continues and the patient's circulatory status is deteriorating even with treatment, surgery is indicated. Obviously, if urine leakage is seen on IVP, surgery is necessary.

Partial or total nephrectomy is indicated if severe parenchymal damage has occurred. The surgeon must remember to visually evaluate and palpate the opposite kidney before nephrectomy. When renal damage is suspected, a preoperative intravenous pyelogram is mandatory to determine the extent and location of the damage and to evaluate the normal kidney and ureters. Renal function should be closely monitored postoperatively. Diuretics (e.g., mannitol or furosemide) may be required if urine production is not adequate.

Ureteral damage causes leakage of urine into the retroperitoneal space. Intraperitoneal urine can be present if the peritoneum has also been disrupted. The ureters may be torn, crushed, or avulsed from the kidney or bladder. Ureteral leakage should be suspected when retroperitoneal fluid is seen radiographically, and urine production is below normal. An IVP is necessary to delineate the ureteral tear, and should always be done preoperatively when this type of injury is suspected. Ureteral damage can be difficult to identify in surgery if an IVP has not been performed. The retroperitoneal tissues are edematous, hemorrhagic, and surrounded by fluid, hampering visibility. Small catheters (Tomcat) or silastic tubing can be passed up the ureters from within the bladder to help identify torn areas. Ureteral tears should be repaired or anastomoses performed using fine sutures (e.g., 5-0, 6-0 Vicryl or Dexon). A stent tube should be placed within the ureter and passed out the urethra. The tube is removed in 5–7 days. Small ureteral tears can be managed with stent tubing alone. A repeat IVP is indicated 4–6 weeks postoperatively to assess ureteral size and to determine whether strictures have resulted from the healing process.

Ureters avulsed from the bladder should be reimplanted using a method similar to that used in reimplanting an ectopic ureter. The ureter is tunneled through the bladder wall near the trigone, and the ureteral mucosa is sutured to the bladder mucosa with 4-0 or 5-0 absorbable suture (Vicryl or Dexon).

Some authors stress that the length of the tunneled portion of ureter must not be excessive to avoid postoperative hydroureter.[17]

The urinary bladder is commonly ruptured with blunt trauma. Bladder tears can occur in any area, but in the authors' experience most have been present on the dorsal surface.

Bladder rupture should be suspected when the bladder cannot be palpated or seen radiographically, and abdominal fluid is present. Extensive inguinal bruising may be present with bladder or urethral tears. Abdominocentesis or DPL may recover urine from the abdomen. Very high creatinine levels in the abdominal fluid are suggestive of uroperitoneum.[4] Positive contrast cystography is the definitive test for a ruptured bladder. A retrograde urethrogram–cystogram is a rapid method of assessing both the urethra and the bladder.

Uroperitoneum usually results in increased BUN, creatinine, potassium, and phosphorus serum levels, and decreased sodium and chloride.[4] Dehydration occurs due to massive fluid shifts into the peritoneal cavity.

Surgery should not be performed immediately on patients with ruptured bladder, unless other life-threatening injuries are present. Initial treatment with intravenous fluids, abdominal drains, broad-spectrum antibiotics, and an indwelling urinary catheter is indicated. A tube cystostomy is an effective means of maintaining bladder drainage. A Foley catheter is placed into the bladder through a flank incision. The bladder wall adjacent to the tube is then sutured to the peritoneum to prevent urine leakage into the abdomen. The patient is allowed to stabilize for several hours. Surgical repair of the bladder can then be performed.

Urethral tears, depending upon location, can cause uroperitoneum or subcutaneous urine leakage. Severe bruising of the skin is seen when subcutaneous urine leakage occurs. Primary repair of the urethra is often difficult due to poor tissue viability. A stent urethral catheter in conjunction with abdominal drains or tube cystostomy should be used. Urine output should be monitored via a closed collection system.

Gastrointestinal Tract

The stomach is not commonly injured by abdominal trauma, but the intestines frequently are damaged, especially by penetrating trauma. Puncture of the bowel causes spillage of intestinal contents, and peritonitis rapidly follows. Avulsion of the mesentery from the intestine can occur, causing ischemia of the involved intestinal segment. Necrosis of the tissue will then result in septic peritonitis.

The diagnosis of intestinal perforation can be obtained by several methods. Diagnostic peritoneal lavage will reveal foreign material such as vegetable fibers or muscle fibers on microscopic examination. Plain film radiographs may show free gas in the abdomen. Contrast studies of the intestine reveal the leaking areas. Water soluble contrast agents (Gastrografin) should be used if leakage is suspected.

Intestinal ischemia and necrosis due to mesenteric avulsion causes a delayed peritonitis due to gradual necrosis of the intestinal wall. The patient may initially look stable, but gradually develops vomiting, bloody stool, and intense abdominal pain 2–4 days post-trauma.[9] Signs of ileus and peritonitis are seen on radiographs.

Immediate laparotomy is indicated if intestinal injury is suspected. Delay of surgery only enhances the potential for peritonitis and sepsis. Intestinal perforations should either be debrided and closed, or the segment should be resected. Multiple, large perforations that are close together are best handled by resection and anastomosis. Avulsion of more than a few centimeters of mesentery from the bowel is treated by resection of the ischemic intestinal segment. Mesenteric rents should be closed to avoid strangulation of bowel. Abdominal lavage is indicated if contamination has occurred. Drains, such as sump drains, are placed to allow postoperative lavage and drainage if peritonitis is present. These drains should be left in place for 3–5 days, depending upon the progress of the patient. Systemic antibiotics are administered based upon the results of culture samples obtained during surgery.

Pancreas

Pancreatic injury associated with abdominal trauma is rare. Traumatic pancreatitis associated with falls from high-rise buildings has been reported in cats.[21] The onset of clinical signs associated with this type of injury is delayed (until 3–5 days postinjury). Abdominal pain and a palpable cranial ventral abdominal mass are the initial findings. Radiographically, a mottled density is evident in the cranial–ventral abdomen. If untreated, diffuse peritonitis results. The above clinical and radiographic signs in conjunction with elevated serum lipase levels suggest pancreatic injury and the release of enzymes. Laparotomy should be performed to assess the damage.

Areas of fat saponification are frequently seen after pancreatic injury and pancreatitis. Nonviable areas of pancreas should be resected. Ideally, avulsed pancreatic ducts should be reimplanted. However, this is technically very difficult. Ligation of the duct can also be performed. If accessory ducts remain intact, exocrine function will be maintained. If all ducts are damaged and major portions of the pancreas must be resected, preservation of at least some pancreatic tissue will help to preserve endocrine function. The surgeon must be familiar with the blood supply to the pancreas and duodenum in order to prevent causing duodenal ischemia during pancreatectomy.

Abdominal lavage should be performed before closure, and sump drains should be implanted. The animal should not be fed for 2–3 days postoperatively. Parenteral nutrition or a jejunostomy feeding tube implanted during surgery can be used to maintain postoperative nutrition.[16] A low fat diet should then be offered in small amounts to minimize release of pancreatic lipase.

Uterus

Abdominal trauma can cause rupture of the uterus if the organ is enlarged at the time of the trauma. A ruptured pyometra causes acute peritonitis and endotoxemia and leads to rapid death if not promptly treated. Tearing of uterine vessels can cause severe blood loss and shock. Rupture of a gravid uterus also causes peritonitis.

Uterine damage is usually best treated by ovariohysterectomy. Abdominal lavage should be performed, and drains may be necessary, depending on the degree of contamination.

Abdominal Hernias

Tearing of the abdominal wall can occur from blunt trauma or penetrating trauma such as bite wounds. Common areas affected are the flank, inguinal region, and prepubic region.

The hernias are usually palpable, especially if abdominal organs are present within the hernia. Radiographs are helpful in showing discontinuity of the abdominal wall and herniation of organs, if present.

Surgical repair of hernias can be challenging. Large defects may require synthetic mesh implants (e.g., Marlex) for reconstruction. These materials should be available to the surgeon before doing the procedure. What appears clinically to be a small, simple hernia may actually require extensive reconstruction.

Heavily contaminated hernias such as those resulting from bite wounds should be cleaned, debrided, and treated as an open wound for 3–5 days before repair of the defect. Padded bandages are used to cover the wound and to provide support. This will allow the acute inflammatory response to diminish and allow the patient to recover from the trauma before a major operation is performed. Obviously, if evisceration has occurred or if there is evidence of intra-abdominal injury, laparotomy should be performed promptly.

REFERENCES

1. Ballinger WF, Rutherford RB, Zuidema GD: The Management of Trauma. WB Saunders, Philadelphia, 1968
2. Bjorling DE, Crowe DT, Kolata RJ, Rawlings CA: Penetrating abdominal wounds in dogs and cats. J Am Anim Hosp Assoc 18:742, 1982
3. Brace JJ, Bellhorn T: The history and physical examination of the trauma patient. Vet Clin North Am 10:533, 1980
4. Burrows CF, Bovee KC: Metabolic changes due to experimentally induced rupture of the canine urinary bladder. Am J Vet Res 35:1083, 1974
5. Burt JK, Root CR: Radiographic manifestations of abdominal trauma. J Am Anim Hosp Assoc 7:328, 1971
6. Crane SW: Evaluation and management of abdominal trauma in the dog and cat. Vet Clin North Am 10:655, 1980

7. Crowe DT, Crane SW: Diagnostic abdominal paracentesis and lavage in the evaluation of abdominal injuries in dogs and cats: Clinical and experimental investigations. J Am Vet Med Assoc 168:700, 1976

8. Cox EF: Blunt abdominal trauma—a five-year analysis of 870 patients requiring celiotomy. Ann Surg 199:467, 1984

9. Dorn AS, Hufford TJ, Anderson NV: Four cases of traumatic intestinal injuries in dogs. J Am Anim Hosp Assoc 11:786, 1975

10. Freeark, RJ: Penetrating wounds of the abdomen. N Engl J Med 291:185, 1974

11. Kolata RJ: Abdominal trauma. Comp Cont Ed 1:445, 1979

12. Kolata RJ: Diagnostic abdominal paracentesis and lavage: Experimental and clinical evaluations in the dog. J Am Vet Med Assoc 168:697, 1976

13. Kolata RJ, Johnston DE: Motor vehicle accidents in urban dogs: A study of 600 cases. J Am Vet Med Assoc 167:938, 1975

14. Lowe RJ, Saletta JD, Read DR, Radhakrishnan J, Moss GS: Should laparotomy be mandatory or selective in gunshot wounds of the abdomen. J Trauma 17:903, 1977

15. Madding GF, Lim RC, Kennedy PA: Hepatic and vena caval injuries. Surg Clin North Am 57:275, 1977

16. Page CP, Carlton PK, Andrassy RJ, Feldtman RW, Shield CF: Safe, cost-effective postoperative nutrition—defined formula diet via needle-catheter jejunostomy. Am J Surg 138:939, 1979

17. Rawlings CA: Repair of ectopic ureter. In Bojrab MJ (ed): Current Techniques in Small Animal Surgery, Lea & Febiger, Philadelphia, 1983

18. Rodriguez A, DuPriest RW, Shatney CH: Recognition of intra-abdominal injury in blunt trauma victims. Am Surg 48:456, 1982

19. Spencer CP, Ackerman N: Thoracic and abdominal radiography of the trauma patient. Vet Clin North Am 10:541, 1980

20. Suter PF, Olsson S: The diagnosis of injuries to the intestines, gall bladder and bile ducts in the dog. J Small Anim Pract 11:575, 1970

21. Suter PF, Olsson S: Traumatic hemorrhagic pancreatitis in the cat: A report with emphasis on the radiological diagnosis. J Am Vet Radiol Soc 10:4, 1969

22. Thompson JS, Moore EE, Van Duzer-Moore S, Moore JB, Galloway AC: The evolution of abdominal stab wound management. J Trauma 20:478, 1980

8 | Nontraumatic Surgical Emergencies of the Abdomen

Gary W. Ellison

The patient presenting with an acute abdominal crisis offers the clinician a challenging diagnostic and therapeutic dilemma. The decision of whether or not to explore the abdominal cavity often causes consternation for the small animal practitioner. Most clinicians have experienced the unfortunate case where an incorrect decision was made, resulting in the death of the patient. The purpose of this chapter is to provide a systematic approach for the diagnosis and treatment of nontraumatic surgical emergencies of the abdomen. A basic understanding of the pathophysiology coupled with early diagnosis and state-of-the-art surgical management will hopefully increase our success with these demanding emergencies.

ORIGINS AND PATHOPHYSIOLOGY OF ABDOMINAL PAIN

Noxious stimuli of the abdominal viscera cause direct stimulation of type C fibers that are found in smooth muscle, peritoneum, and mesentery.[13] Visceral pain impulses travel through the splanchnic nerves (sympathetic), splanchnic ganglion, and sympathetic chain before synapsing in the spinal cord via the white rami communicantes. Most of the abdominal viscera receive innervation from both sides of the spinal cord. Because of this multisegmental innervation overlap and spinal cord modulation, visceral abdominal pain is poorly localized and is often perceived as a dull midline burning sensation.

Nerve endings of pain fibers are located in the submucosa and muscularis of the hollow viscus organs (gastrointestinal tract, gall-bladder, and urinary bladder). Consequently, any process that causes fluid or gaseous distention (intestinal obstruction), forceful contraction (hypersegmentation), or traction (adhesions) may produce pain. In the kidney, liver, and prostate, nerve endings are located in the organ capsule, and any stretching of these secondary to acute parenchymal disease causes pain.

The sensory fibers of parietal pain also travel via C nerve fibers which are carried in somatic sensory nerves and reach the thoracolumbar spinal cord at levels corresponding to specific dermatomes. Therefore, parietal pain is more easily point sensitive and, if local in nature, can be correlated to one side or the other.

Inflammation, whether it be secondary to peritonitis or tissue ischemia, will produce abdominal pain by releasing tissue proteinases or vasoactive substances that stimulate nerve endings. The inflammatory response must involve multiple nerve endings and be of an acute nature in order to create visceral abdominal pain. The plentiful nerve endings located in the parietal peritoneum are more sensitive to a massive inflammatory response and this is why the splinted rigid abdominal posture and resistance to palpation is seen in most cases of generalized peritonitis.

ACUTE GASTRIC DILATATION-VOLVULUS (GDV)

Incidence/Clinical Signs

Acute gastric dilatation-volvulus is a life-threatening syndrome that requires prompt recognition and aggressive medical and surgical therapy. Large or giant breed deep-chested dogs are most frequently affected, but the disease is also seen in uncharacteristic breeds such as the Pekingese and Dachshund and has also been reported in the cat.[58] Most dogs are mature or middle-aged, and males are twice as likely to be affected as females.[3]

Patients often demonstrate hypersalivation or retching on presentation. Cranial abdominal distention is usually profound, and tympany is usually demonstrable on blunt percutaneous percussion, especially of the right anterior quadrant. The distended abdomen makes palpation of individual structures difficult. Hyperpnea or dyspnea accompanied by openmouthed breathing may be seen as a function of hypoxia due to diminished diaphragmatic excursion. Circulatory hypoperfusion (shock) is common, as evidenced by pale mucous membranes, prolonged capillary perfusion, tachycardia, and weak rapid femoral pulse. Septic shock may be a factor as well.

Pathophysiology

A lack of good muscle tone of the stomach wall and laxity of the gastrohepatic ligament may contribute to the development of GDV.[61] Gastric dilatation precedes gastric volvulus. Food and fluid distension from overeating or gaseous distension from aerophagia causes abnormal angulation or twisting of the lower esophageal sphincter that prevents belching or vomiting and results in gastric dilatation. As the stomach enlarges, the dilated gastric fundus becomes displaced from a left dorsal to a right ventral position in the abdomen. The pylorus, which normally lies in the right ventral position, moves to the left and craniodorsally where it takes a mid-dorsal position, thereby creating a gastric volvulus. The spleen follows the greater curvature of the stomach to the right. The splenic attachments to the stomach, namely the gastrosplenic ligament and short gastric arteries, lie within the greater omentum and are often torn during the movement of the gastric fundus. Splenomegaly results from venous occlusion or thrombosis of the splenic veins. Vascular lesions are often found on the greater curvature of the stomach and range from fundic hyperemia to full thickness necrosis and perforation where the short gastric vessels have been damaged.[61]

As the stomach dilates, it exerts pressure on the caudal vena cava. Gastric rotation actively occludes the portal vein. Splanchnic visceral congestion, decreased venous return to the right side of the heart, and sequestration of gastric fluids result in a hypovolemic shock. Portal venous occlusion may also initiate endotoxic shock in dogs as a result of failure of the liver to detoxify endotoxins produced in the intestinal tract.[61] Hypotension and a decreased rate of tissue perfusion are conducive to the development of sludging and the occurrence of disseminated intravascular coagulation (DIC). With the increase in intragastric pressure, venous and lymphatic occlusion occur, resulting in tissue hypoxia that may lead to ischemia and necrosis. Neurologic damage to the ganglion cells of Auerbach's plexus may occur, contributing to decreased peristaltic activity, hypotonia, and flaccidity of the patient's stomach. The dilated stomach limits diaphragmatic excursions, causing decreased tidal volume. The patient compensates by increasing the respiratory rate to maintain adequate minute volume.

Diagnosis

An accurate diagnosis of acute gastric dilatation can usually be made based on signalment, history and physical exam findings. Abdominal radiographs may be performed but are usually delayed until after shock therapy and gastric decompression. With gastric dilatation, the grossly distended gas- and fluid-filled stomach occupies the cranial half of the abdominal cavity pushing remaining abdominal viscera caudally. The spleen is often not visible in its normal location and sometimes is displaced more to the right and dorsally. Evidence of gastric volvulus is suspected when the pylorus is located dorsally and cranially and has shifted to the left of the midline. After gastric decompression the radiographic appearance varies considerably. The stomach may appear in a classic "upside down" configuration, with the fundus located ventrally and the pylorus located dorsally on the lateral projection. In some cases the stomach may remain malpositioned for days without functional disturbance.[20]

Preoperative Management

Since gastric dilatation merely precedes gastric volvulus, the two conditions should be managed similarly: (1) shock therapy, (2) gastric decompression, and (3) monitoring of cardiac dysrhythmias are the primary preoperative goals in the management of GDV. Patient survival often depends on rapid intravenous infusion of large volumes of isotonic fluid. If endotoxic shock is suspected, appropriate antibiotics and corticosteroid therapy are instituted.

Gastric decompression is attempted via orogastric catheterization using a well lubricated polyethylene plastic foal stomach tube. The tube is measured from the mouth to the 13th rib and marked with adhesive tape to assure proper length. The tube is passed with the aid of a mouth gag or through a roll of adhesive tape placed in the dog's mouth. Resistance is met at the gastroesophageal junction, but passage is evident when an abrupt reflux of gas and fluid occurs. When tube passage is difficult, an assistant places the patient in an upright (sitting) position by supporting the dog at the elbows. This sometimes causes the stomach to drop away from the diaphragm enough to allow tube passage. *Ability to pass the stomach tube does not mean that gastric volvulus is not present.* Passage of the tube is possible with a greater than 180° volvulus.[62] If tube passage is not possible, trocharization (gastrocentesis) is performed in the right paracostal area with a 16–18-gauge needle. Trocharization should not be attempted prior to gastric intubation because of the risks for gastric laceration and the limited ability to decompress the stomach. Partial removal of gastric air often allows passage of the gastric tube. After intubation, the gastric contents are removed with multiple saline or warm water lavages. This can be accomplished using a funnel with gravity flow, a large animal dose syringe, or a stomach pump.

Electrocardiographic monitoring of the patient is essential for detection of cardiac dysrhythmias commonly associated with GDV. Myocardial hypoxia caused by the hypotensive shock are the probable cause of the ventricular dysrhythmias. Cardiac dysrhythmias are not always evident on initial presentation but often become apparent within 24 hours. They are a common problem in the postoperative period and require critical early monitoring. Lidocaine, procainamide, and quinidine have all been successfully used to manage GDV-associated tachycardias.

Operative Management of Gastric Dilatation-Volvulus

Patients with GDV will almost always require surgical intervention. Decompression and stabilization alone will result in up to an 80 percent recurrence rate of the disease.[63] Difficulty comes in establishing when to operate and what type of procedure to perform. Some advocate waiting days or even weeks after the initial insult to perform derotation and prophylactic gastropexy. Follow-up results have shown significant mortality associated with fundic necrosis when using this approach.[21]

The author advocates an exploratory laparotomy as soon as the patient is assessed to be a reasonable anesthetic risk. This allows early derotation of the stomach and evaluation of gastric wall viability. Devitalized areas of the stomach can be detected early, and partial gastrectomy may be necessary. If resection is not done, prophylactic gastropexy is performed. If tissue ischemia is extensive and resection is impossible, the animal can be euthanatized and spared the morbidity associated with an inevitable full thickness necrosis, perforation, and death.

Temporary Procedures

If cardiac dysrhythmias or shock prevent an early surgical intervention, a temporary measure can be undertaken. A pharyngostomy tube or gastrostomy procedure can be performed to maintain gastric decompression while stabilizing the patient. Laparotomy and prophylactic gastropexy can then be performed on an elective basis.

The use of pharyngostomy tubes should be reserved for cases that will be operated on within a relatively short period of time, because of their tendency to occlude with resultant continued gastric distention. Once the orogastric tube has been passed, conversion to a pharyngostomy tube is easily performed, but this usually requires narcotic analgesia or general anesthesia. Care must be taken to assure proper tube placement, and postoperative radiographs are indicated. Tubes positioned in the distal esophagus will not facilitate gastric decompression, and those that are too long may result in pressure necrosis along the greater curvature of the stomach. Periodic flushing of the tube with water is required in order to help to assure its patency.

Cutaneous gastrostomy can usually be performed with an inverted "L" block of 2 percent lidocaine or other local analgesic in the right paracostal area.[45] A 5 cm vertical incision is made through the skin and subcutaneous tissue 5 cm caudal to the 13th rib and 15 cm lateral to the midline. A grid incision is carried sequentially down through the external oblique, internal oblique, and transverse abdominis muscles to the peritoneum. The distended gastric fundus pouches into the incision, once the peritoneum is incised. The exact orientation of the stomach is difficult to determine, and derotation of the stomach is not attempted. The stomach wall is secured at the dorsal and ventral aspects of the peritoneum with two simple interrupted sutures of 2-0 nylon. The seromuscular layer of the stomach is then sutured to the peritoneum with a simple continuous layer of 2-0 nylon around the periphery of the incision. Care is taken to create a tight seal that prevents any leakage into the peritoneal cavity. A stab incision is then made into the stomach lumen and extended to a 4 cm length. Submucosa and mucosa are then sutured to the skin with simple interrupted 2-0 nylon sutures, completing the 2-layer closure. The stomach can then be lavaged or suctioned through the gastrostomy stoma. Petrolatum is liberally applied around the gastrostomy site to prevent skin irritation from developing secondary to gastric reflux. Closure of the gastrostomy site is made in reverse order. After removing the skin sutures, the mucosa and submucosa are inverted using a continuous Cushing pattern, followed by a continuous Lembert pattern in the serosa and muscularis. 2-0 Polyglycolic acid or polyglactin 910 is used. The continuous suture pattern approximating the stomach and peritoneum is cut, and the stomach drops away from the peritoneum. The grid incision is closed with interrupted sutures in each of the three muscle bellies, followed by routine closure of the subcutaneous tissue and skin. Further examination of the gastrotomy site for quality of closure is made during exploratory laparotomy of the abdomen.

Intra-abdominal Management of GDV

Definitive surgical management of GDV involves (1) repositioning of the stomach and spleen and, (2) a prophylactic procedure to prevent recurrence. Ancillary procedures that may be necessary include a splenectomy or some form of pyloric surgery.

Upon exploration of the abdomen, the stomach is covered on its ventral surface by omentum. The stomach usually rotates clockwise when the dog is viewed from behind. The stomach is derotated from the left side of the table. The right hand is passed along the left abdominal wall and the pylorus is located in its left dorsal position. It is derotated in a counterclockwise position to its normal right ventral position. Counterclockwise rotations are handled in an opposite manner to that of clockwise rotations. The spleen is returned to its normal position and anatomically realigned. Moderate to severe splenomegaly is usually evident. Initial examination of the splenic vessels for thrombosis is performed. Splenomegaly due to venous occlusion will usually not resolve completely during the course of the surgical procedure. If good arterial pulsations are present without evidence of arterial thrombosis or avulsion of vessels, the spleen should be retained. Occasionally thrombosis or avulsion of the splenic vessels with subsequent infarction necessitates splenectomy.

The stomach is examined for viability and necrosis in the area of the greater curvature of the fundus, extending to the cardia. Differentiating viable from necrotic tissue is sometimes difficult, as sharp lines of demarcation are not always evident. Since gastric atony is usually profound, and gastric contractions are poor, determination of viability is usually made by tissue color and palpation. A viable gastric wall varies from pink to dark red or is hyperemic in appearance and has a normal thickness. Nonviable tissue is dark blue to black and characteristic thinning of the gastric wall is evident on palpation.

The necessity for gastric outflow surgery is controversial. Pyloric surgery has been advocated by some to relieve gastric retention and accelerate gastric emptying.[61] Delayed gastric emptying as a cause of gastric dilatation-volvulus has been hypothesized but not conclusively proven in the dog. Mucosal and submucosal hemorrhage and edema associated with GDV have been documented (Moore RW, Colorado State University, 1981). These acute lesions were felt to be caused by twisting of the stomach rather than by primary lesions. Since the role of pyloric obstruction is questionable in GDV, the extra time and danger to the patient from pyloric surgery is only warranted if there is a history of gastric outflow obstruction or if gross palpation of the pylorus at surgery indicates the presence of disease.

Pyloromyotomy (Fredret–Ramstedt), pyloroplasty (Heineke–Mickulicz), or Y–U antral advancement flaps are all procedures that may be used to relieve pyloric outflow obstruction. The superiority of one technique over the other in increasing gastric outflow has not been well established in the dog. With this in mind, the pyloromyotomy technique is safest, as it does not involve entering the bowel lumen. However, a major disadvantage to the pyloromyotomy is that gastric outflow obstruction due to mucosal hypertrophy may not be detected by this technique. Pyloric obstructions of this etiology need to be corrected with one of the open surgical techniques.

Numerous surgical techniques have been described for the prevention of GDV recurrence. Variations of permanent gastropexies and tube gastrostomies have been most popular in recent years.[37,44] We currently use and prefer the circumcostal gastropexy.[18] The advantages of the circumcostal gastropexy are (1) the speed and simplicity of the technique, (2) better anatomical alignment of the stomach, (3) the stomach lumen is not entered, thereby alleviating the possibility of leakage and peritonitis, and (4) postoperative convalescence time has been reduced. Also, a recent study has shown that circumcostal gastropexies have a stronger adhesion that does not decrease in strength with time when compared with other techniques (Fox S Ellison G, University of Florida, 1984).

Postoperative Care

Postoperative management of the GDV patient primarily involves fluid and electrolyte therapy as well as continuous cardiac monitoring. Postoperative hypokalemia is common and is managed by intravenous potassium supplementation (20 mEq/L). Once oral alimentation occurs, the hypokalemia usually resolves. Monitoring of cardiac dysrhythmias is sometimes required for up to one week postoperatively.

When utilizing the circumcostal gastropexy, the patients are fed small amounts of baby food the day following surgery. The diet is gradually increased in amount over a 10-day period. Gastritis resolves rapidly, and vomiting has been rare beyond 24 hours in patients without gastric resection. Discharge is determined by the patient's postoperative cardiac status, but commonly animals are released 3–4 days following surgery. Postoperative antibiotics are generally reserved for cases in which partial gastrectomy, gastrotomy, or peritoneal contamination was present, but are not used in uncomplicated cases.

INTESTINAL OBSTRUCTION

Etiology

In the dog, the oropharyhgeal opening is larger than any other opening aborally. Obstruction may occur along any site distal to this opening. Foreign bodies cause most intestinal obstructions, and careful questioning of the owner will sometimes disclose the source. Common objects include bones, rubber balls, cellophane wrappers, and corn cobs. Linear foreign bodies are a common cause of obstruction in the cat. Other causes of acute intestinal obstruction include intestinal volvulus, intussusceptions, and incarcerations.

History/Clinical Signs

Clinical signs are dependent on the level (high, low) and the degree of the obstruction (partial, complete). Vomiting is usually reported in the history. With high (pylorus, duodenum, proximal jejunum) and complete obstructions, vomiting is often projectile and unrelenting in nature. Rapid fluid and electrolyte changes with subsequent dehydration may result. With distal intestinal obstruction (jejunum, ileum, colon) vomiting is often reported early in the course but anorexia and bowel distention follow. Complete obstruction created experimentally in the mid-jejunum in dogs resulted in vomiting that occurred after 24–36 hours and then decreased to once a day. These dogs were able to survive for several weeks, as long as free choice water was available.[17]

Careful questioning of the owner may help in establishing the level of obstruction. Bilious vomitus suggests that the lesion is distal to the bile duct, whereas feculent vomitus suggests a distal bowel obstruction. Slow-moving foreign bodies may historically manifest clinical characteristics of both types of vomitus.

Incomplete obstructions caused by intraluminal linear foreign bodies or neoplasia usually present with a chronic insidious course with sporadic vomiting and/or cachexia. The clinical course often progresses over days or weeks. Conversely, complete obstructions caused by foreign bodies, incarcerated intestines, acute intussusceptions, or intestinal volvulus usually cause acute bowel distention with unrelenting clinical signs.

The presence and character of feces is sometimes important in establishing the type of obstruction. Scanty stools often indicate an incomplete obstruction (as is often seen in young animals with intussusception) or may represent residual fecal material present prior to the obstruction. Melena may indicate intestinal strangulation, ulcerations, neoplasia, or parasitism. Diarrhea, tenesmus, and/or scanty amounts of bloodstained feces are often seen in patients with intussusception.

Pathophysiology of Intestinal Obstruction

Experimental and clinical data support the fact that animals with small intestinal obstruction that vomit profusely survive for a shorter period of time than those that do not vomit. More than half of all the fluids and electrolytes are secreted in the stomach and duodenum, and the majority of these are reabsorbed by the jejunum and ileum.[54] Distal duodenal obstruction prevents large quantities of salivary, gastric, pancreatic secretions, or oral fluids from contacting the jejunal and ileal mucosal surfaces for reabsorption. Obstruction of the distal small intestine spares most of the absorptive surface. Electrolyte loss is closely associated with and dependent upon the level of obstruction. With obstructions at the pylorus, gastric fluids rich in potassium (K^+), sodium (Na^+), hydrogen (H^+), and chloride (Cl^-) ions are vomited, and a hypochloremic, hypokalemic, moderately hyponatremic, metabolic alkalosis with dehydration may result.[33] Most obstructions distal to the bile and pancreatic ducts will result in loss of highly alkaline duodenal, pancreatic, and biliary secretions. Metabolic acidosis usually results from loss of these bicarbonate-rich duodenal contents.

Dilation of the intestine proximal to the obstruction is a well-recognized phenomenon. Regardless of the etiology, inhibition of motility and accumulation of air and fluid within the lumen of the bowel occurs. Gaseous distention proximal to the obstruction is mainly due to swallowed air, although some diffusion from the blood may occur. Fluid distention results in increased bowel secretion and decreased reabsorption from the gut mucosa.[39] This sequestration of fluid within the bowel lumen coupled with loss due to emesis is responsible for the profound extracellular dehydration and hypovolemia that may be seen in cases of complete bowel obstruction.[49]

Adynamic (Paralytic) Ileus

Adynamic (paralytic) ileus or nonobstructive bowel distention has been used to describe a variety of conditions that result in an inability of the intestine to propulse ingesta, in spite of the lack of mechanical obstruction.[54] Gas and fluid fill the lumen and produce distention of the bowel similar to that seen with true obstruction. Adynamic ileus is a major problem in humans following abdominal surgery. Intra-abdominal trauma, peritonitis, and anticholinergic drug therapy are other common causes. Ileus is probably an overdiagnosed finding in small animal medicine and surgery. Radiographic signs associated with large, dilated loops of bowel are most often associated with mechanical obstruction in small animal patients. However, when adynamic ileus is felt to be present, it should be treated by bowel decompression, fluid and electrolyte support, treatment of existing sepsis, and removal of the cause.

Simple Mechanical Versus Strangulated (Ischemic) Obstruction

Distinguishing between simple mechanical and strangulated (ischemic) bowel obstruction is critical, because the latter condition requires early and rapid surgical intervention. Mechanical obstructions can be luminal (foreign bodies), intramural (neoplasia), or extramural (adhesions). With simple mechanical luminal obstruction, blood flow to the distended bowel is not completely obliterated, but increased bowel wall tension may cause both histologic

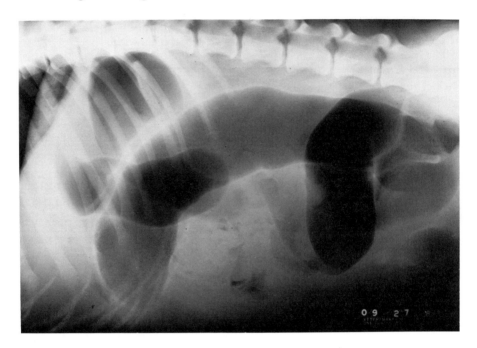

Fig. 8-1. Lateral abdominal radiograph of an ileocecal intussusception. Note the large, fixed, dilated loops of bowel.

and physiologic changes. Venous and lymphatic hydrostatic pressures are elevated initially, while arterial pressures do not result in vascular compromise. Reduced capillary flow, diminished tissue perfusion, and the subsequent increase in vascular permeability result in extravasation of fluid into the interstitium. Intramural edema can become severe enough to result in diminished blood flow, resulting in hypoxia, tissue ischemia, and mucosal necrosis.

Strangulated obstruction may occur from intraluminal obstruction due to local pressure necrosis and subsequent perforation of the bowel. More commonly, strangulation obstruction occurs secondarily to mesenteric vascular disruption caused by intestinal volvulus (Fig. 8-1), intussusception, or strangulation hernia. Primary vascular disease leading to thromboembolism and secondary ischemia, as seen in human beings and horses, is an uncommon finding in small animals.

In strangulated forms of obstruction, the metabolically active mucosa is extremely sensitive to insufficient profusion and anoxia and therefore undergoes necrosis quickly. After the mucosal barrier is destroyed, bacteria and endotoxins pass transmurally into the lymphatics and peritoneal cavity where they are absorbed into the systemic circulation. Vasoactive properties of bacteria, endotoxins, and free peritoneal hemoglobin create the systemic hypotension and septic shock that make strangulation obstruction so lethal.

DIAGNOSIS OF THE EMERGENCY OBSTRUCTION/ PERFORATION

Physical Exam

Physical diagnosis of small intestinal obstruction by palpation will shorten the diagnostic process and hasten surgical correction. Careful examination of the ventral abdomen for painful and nonreducible umbilical or inguinal hernias may indicate incarceration of a segment of bowel. The animal's forelimbs are raised to facilitate palpation of the anterior abdomen. Skillful palpation may be critical in determining an elusive foreign body or pleated segments of bowels. A mid-abdominal to caudally located longitudinal circular mass may represent a classic "sausage shaped" ileocecal intussusception. Abdominal distention or splinting may be indicative of peritonitis. Presumptive diagnosis of peritonitis can be made if there is evidence of peritoneal fluid associated with abdominal pain in the presence of a fever. Radiography and diagnostic peritoneal lavage are necessary to confirm the diagnosis.

Radiography

An easily diagnosed radiopaque foreign body will occasionally, but not usually, be associated with an acute abdominal emergency. Many times, the etiology of the obstruction cannot be determined, but diagnosing it as complete or incomplete, proximal or distal is useful to the surgeon. Radiographic signs characteristic of simple obstruction, strangulation obstruction, or perforation are more important in determining rapid surgical intervention than is a specific diagnosis.

Gas and fluid distention of the small intestine are usually present with complete intestinal obstruction. Air-capped fluid lines of different levels are sometimes demonstrable on a standing lateral view. Radiographic evidence of complete intestinal obstruction, coupled with palpable foreign bodies, intussusceptions, or incarcerated hernias, are all indications for surgery. Nonemergency causes of gaseous or fluid distention in the bowel are aerophagia, hypotensive crisis (shock), anticholinergic drugs, enemas, postoperative ileus, and peritonitis. The presence of free peritoneal air in the absence of prior abdominal surgery or trocharization is definitive for gastrointestinal perforation. A painful abdomen accompanied by free peritoneal fluid, fever, leukocytosis, or the presence of degenerated PMNs or bacteria on diagnostic peritoneal lavage, indicates the need for an exploratory coeliotomy.

If plain film radiography is nondiagnostic, a contrast study is performed. Barium sulfate may be administered by stomach tube at a dose of 5–8 ml/kg. If perforation is suspected but cannot be confirmed on plain films, an iodinated contrast material may be substituted to reduce the potential for barium-induced peritonitis. The iodides are less effective contrast materials because of the dilution and absorption they undergo in the distal intestine. Also, since they are hyperosmolar compounds, they may lead to progressive dehydration and are contraindicated in animals who are debilitated.

Abnormal findings on the contrast GI study include delayed transit time, narrow lumen, fixed and displaced loops of intestine, and radiolucent foreign bodies. Fixation of a dilated loop of bowel in multiple radiographic projections (i.e., a dilated loop of bowel through a diaphragmatic rent) or an isolated segment of intestine dilated by fluid (intussusception) in conjunction with pain, fever, or depression are indicative that strangulation of the bowel is present.

Diagnostic Paracentesis and Peritoneal Lavage

Diagnostic peritoneal lavage is a clinically reliable technique that has been of great benefit in the diagnosis of intra-abdominal emergencies in man and has been established as an invaluable technique in veterinary institutions. It is a technique that can be easily done in veterinary practice with the same beneficial results. A recent study showed diagnostic lavage to be 95 percent accurate in picking up intra-abdominal injury and disease in 129 dogs and cats, whereas needle paracentesis alone was only 47 percent accurate.[11]

A local lidocaine block is performed 1–2 cm caudal to the umbilicus after a 10 cm square clip and prep. A commercial peritoneal dialysis catheter* or a 14-gauge indwelling intravenous cathether† is directed through the body wall and aspirated for fluid. If no fluid is aspirated, 20 ml/kg of warmed lactated Ringer's or 0.9 percent NaCl solution is infused via gravity flow through a sterile IV infusion set. The fluid is mixed with abdominal contents by gentle abdominal massage and then collected by gravity flow into a sterile receptacle. Ten ml of fluid is sufficient for most diagnostic tests; however, as much of the fluid should be removed as possible to minimize discomfort to the patient.

Laboratory interpretation of the peritoneal lavage fluid should include PCV, leukocyte count, and cytology. Amylase levels, creatinine levels, and bilirubin tests may be diagnostic for intestinal ischemia, pancreatic inflammation, urinary tract leakage, or biliary tract injury, respectively. The interpretation of fluid from diagnostic peritoneal lavage is listed in Table 8-1.

Other Laboratory Tests

A markedly elevated white count due to neutrophilia and a left shift may be caused by a localized peritonitis, inflammation, or bowel wall necrosis. The markedly painful animal may also demonstrate a mature neutrophila and lymphopenia due to a stress leukogram. Commonly, leukopenia with degenerated or toxic neutrophils is seen with acute septic peritonitis or bowel incarceration, along with an elevated PCV and reduced serum glucose.

---

* Trocath, McCaw Laboratories, Div. of American Hospital Corp., Glendale, CA.

† Sovereign Indwelling Catheter, Monoject, Div. of Sherwood Medical, Brunswick Company, St. Louis, MO.

Table 8-1. Interpretation of Fluid in Diagnostic Peritoneal Lavage[1,20]

Test	Significance
WBC Count	1,000/mm^3 is indicative of peritonitis
	2,000/mm^2 is indicative of severe peritonitis
PCV	1% PCV elevation is seen for every 10–20 ml of free blood in abdomen per 500 ml of lavage fluid
Cytology	Many toxic neutrophils indicate supporative peritonitis. Careful examination of neutrophils for intracellular bacteria should be made. The presence of vegetative fibers with free bacteria indicates hollow viscous leakage or disruption.
Amylase	> 1,000 units supporative indicate intestinal ischemia or pancreatic inflammation
Alkaline phosphatase	> serum concentration indicates intestinal ischemia or strangulation
Creatinine	> serum creatine levels indicates the presence of uroperitoneum
Ictotest[a]	Ictotest positive—leakage from the biliary tree

[a] Urine bilirubin test tablets, Ames Division of Miles Laboratories, Inc, Elkhart, IN.

FOREIGN BODIES

Incidence/Clinical Signs

Surgical management of gastrointestinal foreign bodies varies depending on the type and location of the foreign body. Sharp foreign bodies such as straight pins, safety pins, bones, nails, or glass will usually pass through the gastrointestinal tract without creating intestinal perforation. Rubber balls, cellophane, or corn cobs tend to pass slower or not at all and are more likely to cause complete mechanical obstruction requiring emergency laparotomy. Gastric foreign bodies usually cause sporadic vomiting and can be handled on an elective basis unless complete pyloric obstruction is evident.

Treatment

Singular or multiple foreign bodies such as corn cobs that cause complete mechanical obstruction are easily located. In these cases, important decisions must be made regarding bowel viability. With a complete obstruction, intestinal distention proximal to the obstruction is often profound and the distended loops of bowel take on a cyanotic appearance. Intestinal viability is best evaluated after decompressing the dilated loops of bowel and removing the foreign body. Decompression of fluid and gas from the proximal segment of the distended bowel is performed with a 20-gauge needle and suction apparatus or a 60 cc syringe with a three-way stopcock. If intestinal wall ischemia and necrosis is present with dark fetid tissue or perforation and peritonitis, then resection and anastomosis is performed immediately. However, in most cases of simple nonstrangulated obstruction, bowel viability is maintained and the visual appearance of dark, distended, loops of bowel improves rapidly after removal of the insult.

When assessing questionable areas of bowel viability, standard clinical criteria are color, arterial pulsations, and the presence of peristalsis. Of these three parameters, experimental data has shown peristalsis to be the best and most dependable determinant of viability. The "pinch test" should be performed on questionable bowel to determine whether smooth muscle contraction and peristalsis can be initiated. Experimental determination of bowel viability has included temperature probes, pH monitors, a doppler device to monitor blood flow and, most recently, the use of intravenous vital dyes. Of the latter group, fluorescein dye has gained widespread use as a safe, effective, inexpensive, and practical method in both human and veterinary patients to determine gastrointestinal viability.[14,59] Twenty mg/kg of sodium fluorescein dye is given intravenously through any peripheral vein and within a 2-minute period the tissues are subjected to 3,600 Å wave ultraviolet light (Wood's lamp). Normal bowel viability demonstrates a bright green glow with a smooth, uniform fluorescence. Areas of bowel are considered viable if they have a normal or fine granular fluorescent pattern, i.e., a mottled pattern not as bright as normal intestine, but where no areas of nonfluorescence exceed 3 mm in diameter. Areas of bowel are not viable if they have a patchy density where areas of non-fluorescence exceed 3 mm or where there is only perivascular fluorescence if completely non-fluorescent areas are seen.[59]

Enterotomy Techniques

If the involved segment of intestine is viable, an enterotomy is made. After milking intestinal contents 10 cm to either side of the foreign body and packing the intestinal off from the abdominal cavity, the selected bowel is held by the assistant with moistened sponges or Doyen intestinal forceps. A longitudinal incision is made in the antimesenteric border of the intestine in the viable tissue immediately distal to the foreign body. Bright red blood exuding from the cut edge suggests that vascular supply is intact, whereas dark cyanotic blood may indicate that tissue ischemia is present. The foreign body is gently delivered through the enterotomy incision, taking care not to tear the incision margins.

Closure of the enterotomy incision is usually made in a longitudinal fashion. A variety of closure patterns are acceptable. Simple interrupted appositional or crushing patterns have sutures placed 3–4 mm apart and 2–3 mm from the cut edge, taking care to incorporate all layers of the intestinal wall. A modified Gambee pattern incorporates the serosa muscularis and submucosa but excludes most of the mucosa and is helpful in reducing the mucosal eversion that tends to occur. If enterotomy leakage is likely because of a hypoproteinemic or cachexic state, a continuous inverting Cushing, Connell, or Lembert pattern is performed. This provides a more watertight seal and gives good serosa to serosa apposition. Single layer closures are used because double layer closures may cause excessive compromise of the lumen diameter. All suturing is done with 3-0 to 4-0 polyglactin 910, polyglycolic acid or polydioxanone on a taper-cut needle. Chromic catgut has been used with clinical success and is probably safe for use in the small intestine. However, experimental work has documented that it breaks down rapidly in the stomach because of the acidic environment.[15] Also, catgut is not a good choice of suture for use in the colon because of that tissue's slow healing properties and the presence of collagenase that may enhance loss of the tensile strength of the suture.

Linear foreign bodies caused by such items as fishing line, meat wrappers, or sewing yarn present a difficult surgical problem. The trailing end of a string foreign body often becomes tethered to the base of the tongue or the pyloric area of the stomach. Intestinal peristalsis attempts to move the foreign body distally, resulting in bowel plication. The string may cut through the wall on the mesenteric surface, resulting in peritonitis. Linear foreign bodies should be managed by initially identifying and releasing the anchor point. If wrapped around the tongue, the foreign body should be released prior to laparotomy. More commonly, a gastrotomy is necessary to free the wadded string or fish line from its gastropyloric anchor point. Multiple enterotomies are then usually required to facilitate complete removal of the foreign body. If too few enterotomies are made, with too much traction placed on the string, the mesenteric border may be perforated in an area that is difficult to explore and suture. Occasionally the string has cut through at several locations, and peritonitis is evident. Sometimes, in longstanding cases, fibrosis has occurred around the foreign body to such an extent that even after its removal, the bowel retains its pleated conformation. In these cases, intestinal resection and anastomosis may be necessary.

Technique for Intestinal Resection and Anastomosis

When resection and anastomosis is necessary, the mesenteric vessels to the affected bowel are isolated and ligated between ligatures. The arcuate vessels located along the mesenteric boundary are then ligated. At least 1.5 cm of viable tissue is included in the proximal and distal boundaries of the devitalized tissue to be removed. Intestinal contents are milked proximally and distally and held by an assistant with moistened saline-soaked sponges or with Doyen intestinal forceps. Carmalt or other crushing clamps are placed in the area of intestine to be resected at a 60° angle away from the long axis of the intestine. A scalpel blade is used to excise the bowel along the outside of the crushing clamp. The mesentery is then transected and the excised bowel removed from the surgical field. Up to an 80 percent resection of the small intestine is consistent with quality of life.[9] Resections greater than this lead to weight loss, cachexia, macrocytic anemia, hypoproteinemia, and chronic diarrhea.

Differences in luminal diameter sometimes make end-to-end anastomosis difficult. The lumen diameter of the smaller segment can be enlarged by either cutting the tissue back at a more acute angle or making a short incision along its mesenteric border.

A variety of suture patterns have been used successfully for end-to-end intestinal anastomoses in the small animal patient, but at the present time approximating patterns are recommended. Properly performed approximating patterns create an increased lumen diameter when compared to everting or inverting patterns. They also give rapid and precise primary intestinal healing and minimize the potential for postoperative adhesion formation. Everting anastomoses, although initially creating larger lumen diameter, ultimately lead to stenosis of the lumen.[15] Delayed mucosal healing, mucocele formation, prolonged inflammatory response, and increased adhesion formation are all reasons why everting anastomoses are not recommended. Inverting anastomoses have the advantage of being more leak-resistant due to good serosa to serosa contact but create an internal cuff of tissue that may compromise the lumen diameter. If the vascular supply to this internal cuff of tissue strangulates, it will eventually necrose and slough. Inflammation is more severe, and healing time of inverting patterns is delayed when compared to approximating technique. Despite the aforementioned disadvantages, inverting techniques should be considered for use in colonic resection and anastomosis where the high bacterial content of feces makes leakage of the anastomosis extremely dangerous. Simple interrupted approximating and simple interrupted crushing techniques are the most commonly used techniques for approximating end-to-end anastomoses. The crushing suture has been shown to cause more tissue ischemia directly at the suture line but has equal bursting strengths when compared to the approximating technique.[4,14] Eversion of mucosa from the bowel edge can be overcome by sharply incising the mucosa with Metzenbaum scissors or by using a modified Gambee suture pattern. Regardless of the suture technique used, it is critical to secure the submucosa, which is the layer of greatest strength.

The anastomosis is began at the mesenteric border because the presence of fat in this area makes suture placement more difficult. Leakage is more likely to occur at this point. A second suture is placed on the antimesenteric border with the third and fourth sutures placed at the 90 degree quadrants respectively. Two to three more sutures are placed between each of the four quadrant sutures at 3 mm intervals, resulting in a total of 10 to 16 sutures. The anastomosis is checked for leakage by infusing saline under moderate pressure into the intestinal lumen.

After the anastomosis has been completed, the mesenteric defect is closed with a simple continuous pattern, carefully not including the mesenteric vasculature within the sutures. The anastomosis is then covered with a pedicle of greater omentum. The omentum is critical to the successful healing of the intestinal wounds, especially in patients with peritonitis. In one study, 9 to 10 dogs with experimentally induced peritonitis and removal of the omentum died after intestinal anastomosis. When the omentum remained, 10 out of 10 dogs survived.[38]

INTUSSUSCEPTION

Incidence/Clinical Signs

Intussusceptions are most often seen in immature animals. The exact biomechanical cause of the condition is unknown and has not been reproduced experimentally, but some investigators feel that a local incongruency of the intestine caused by induration or spasticity (intestinal parasitism) or sudden diameter change (in the ileocecal area) occurs. A proximal bowel segment then invaginates (intussusceptum) into a distal section of bowel (intussuscipiens).[50] Reverse peristalsis may also play a role in the etiopathogenesis of the condition. Heavy intestinal parasitism with ascarids or coccidia, as well as severe enteritis seen with canine distemper, are reported as predisposing causes. Intussusceptions are also seen with increasing frequency after elective or nonelective exploratory coeliotomies.

Recently, we have seen a high number of cases associated with parvo virus-induced enteritis. Although conclusive studies regarding morbidity and mortality are not available, early experience suggests that these cases carry a more guarded prognosis. Increased mortality of these cases may be due to predisposing fluid and electrolyte imbalances, agranulocytosis and secondary bacterial septicemia, and an increased tendency for the intussusceptions to recurr.

Clinical signs depend on the completeness and level of obstruction. The majority of intussusceptions occur at the ileocolic junction, but higher jejunojejunal or even pylorogastric intussusceptions are reported.[36] Patients with high intussusceptions usually undergo profuse vomiting and rapid dehydration. Ileocolic intussusceptions often present with a history of sporadic vomition, inappetance, or hematotenesmus.

Acuteness or severity of signs also depends on the degree of obstruction. With an acute massive intussusception, vomiting, rapid dehydration and electrolyte imbalance may be seen. In the early stages, venous congestion causes the walls of the intussusceptum to become edematous, turgid and engorged with blood. Acute intussusceptions rapidly become irreducible as a result of the congestion and outpouring of fibrinous exudate from the serosal surfaces. As the blood supply is more completely embarrassed, ischemia and necrosis of the invaginated bowel occurs. Transmural migration of bacterial organisms and endotoxins may evolve into endotoxic shock, rapid cardiovascular collapse, and death.

In most cases, the obstruction is incomplete, and a chronic course of inappetance or bloody tenesmus is seen for several weeks. Although the invaginated bowel may become devitalized, perforation is rare because the outer ensheathing layer retains its viability, and fibrinous adhesions seal the proximal border of the intussusception. Occasionally, spontaneous recovery occurs when the nonviable intussusceptum is sloughed, and patency of the intestinal lumen is reestablished.[60]

Diagnosis

Diagnosis of intussusceptions can usually be accomplished by simple abdominal palpation and radiography (Fig. 8-1). A cylindrical, sausage-shaped mass located in the mid- to caudal abdomen is pathognomonic for the disease.

Treatment

Surgical management of intussusceptions involves reduction and/or resection and anastomosis. Prophylactic enteropexy may be done, as well, to prevent recurrence. Upon identifying the intussusception, it is isolated and packed off from the peritoneal cavity. Reduction is facilitated by gentle milking of the intussusceptum from the intussuscipiens. The ensheathing layer is gently compressed over the apex of the intussusceptum while gentle traction is placed on the proximal segment of bowel. In relatively acute cases, reduction is usually accomplished, and bowel viability is closely scrutinized. When mature adhesions have formed between the invaginated and ensheathing layers, reduction is usually not possible, and resection and anastomosis are performed. In man, resection of the intussuscepted portion of bowel decreases the incidence of occurrence, but, in the dog, no sparing effect has been reported after resection and anastomosis.[60]

Following reduction or resection and anastomosis of the intussusception, a bowel plication or enteropexy technique should be performed. Clinical results with these techniques have been encouraging, although studies documenting their efficacy are not available. Bowel plication involves laying the bowel side by side in a series of gentle loops. At least three loops of plicated bowel are used proximally and three distally to the origin of the intussusception.[16] The loops are sutured together on their antimesenteric border, using simple interrupted sutures of 3-0 to 4-0 nylon or polypropylene (Fig. 8-2). These sutures penetrate the seromuscular layers of bowel but do not enter the lumen.[64] Serosa-to-serosa adhesions form that do not interfere with intestinal motility, barium transit time, or growth rate disturbances.[64] In addition to the bowel plication, an enteropexy can be done. This entails fixing the bowel to the peritoneal surface of the abdominal wall with 4–8 nonabsorbable sutures.

Postoperative Management

Postoperative care of the patient involves fluid and electrolyte support and treatment of the primary cause, if identifiable. Appropriate anthelmintics should be prescribed for endoparasitism and antidiarrheals (kaolin and pectin) for diarrhea. Chemoprophylaxis is used due to the clean–contaminated nature of the surgery. Cefoxitin given intramuscularly (15 mg/kg every 6 hours) for 24 hours before surgery is recommended. If gross spillage is encountered during surgery, then this antibiotic is continued for 5 days. Recurrence of the intussusception is common and usually occurs proximal to the plicated segment of bowel within a few days of the initial surgical repair. Return of vomiting or inappetence usually signals a recurrence and necessitates further surgical repair. The use of anticholinergics postoperatively is controversial at present. Proponents feel that their spasmolytic properties reduce changes of recurrence, whereas opponents feel that they merely contribute to the grossly distended dilated loops of bowel that are often present.

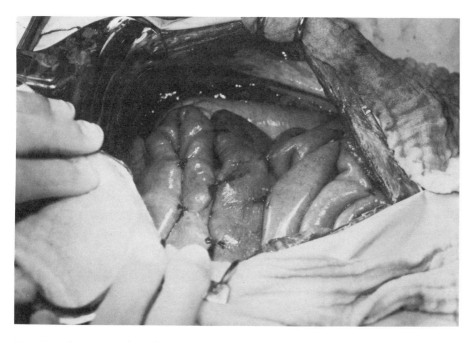

Fig. 8-2. Intraoperative view of an enteropexy technique. Adjacent loops of bowel have been sutured together on their antimesenteric borders with simple interrupted 3-0 catgut sutures. At least three loops of bowel should be plicated proximal and distal to the site of intussusception.

INTESTINAL VOLVULUS

Incidence/Clinical Signs

Intestinal volvulus is defined as the rotation of the bowel around its mesenteric axis (Fig. 8-3). Because of their freely movable unattached mesentery, the jejunum and proximal ileum are the most likely locations for occurrence. Intestinal torsion or rotation of the bowel along its longitudinal axis is uncommonly seen in small animals. Intestinal volvulus is seen primarily in large dogs, greater than 20 kg in weight. There is an approximate 4 to 1 male to female ratio, and the German Shepherd is predisposed.[27]

The proposed etiology of intestinal volvulus in man includes anatomic abnormalities, hereditary predisposition, high fiber diets, and strenuous postprandial exercise. Most dogs present without a prior history of short-term illness. Some patients have diarrhea prior to the onset of signs and, in at least one case, the volvulus was associated with an intestinal tumor. Some cases have undergone an elective or exploratory coeliotomy shortly prior to the episode, suggesting that translocation of the viscera may enter into the etiology of the disease. As with gastric volvulus, these patients undergo a preacute onset of signs and may progress from being normal to near death in less than 6 hours.[27]

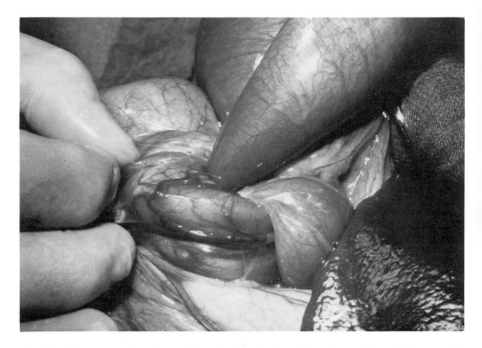

Fig. 8-3. Intraoperative view of intestinal volvulus. Note the twisting of the mesojejunum and incarceration of the bowel wall.

The most common clinical sign is hematochezia, vomiting being very uncommon. Abdominal distention is present in some but not all cases. Intestinal obstruction occurs because of kinking of the bowel at each end of the twisted loop. Bowel distention occurs due to entrapped ingesta and the build-up of fluid and or gas. The combination of obstruction and bowel ischemia results in a rapid production of toxins. Once full-thickness necrosis occurs and significant distention has taken place, the bowel may rupture. If the patient has survived to this point, bacterial peritonitis, endotoxic shock and death will follow rapidly.

Diagnosis

Successful formulation of a diagnosis and early surgical management of intestinal volvulus is essential to the survival of the patient. Mortality is high, with 6 out of 6 dogs dying in one study.[27] Unfortunately, volvulus of the intestine is not associated with characteristic signs. Acute onset of bloody stools, weakness, and collapse may occur within a period of 6 hours. Palpation of multiple turgid dilated loops of bowel in the mid-abdominal region may be suggestive that a volvulus is present. However, accurate palpation is often difficult because of the amount of intestine involved and the secondary abdominal distention.

Clinicopathologic results have been unrewarding. Due to the acute onset, the PCV, WBC counts, and electrolyte values are often near normal. If the animal presents in a hypoperfused state, metabolic acidosis may be evident.

Radiographic diagnosis is difficult because of the many radiographic patterns seen with the disease. Radiographic signs may include gaseous distention of multiple loops of bowel (which are difficult to distinguish from other obstructive patterns), gross distention of the small intestine with ingesta or fecal material, and loss of abdominal detail or ground-glass pattern indicative of peritoneal fluid.

Antemortem diagnosis of intestinal volvulus is made during an exploratory coeliotomy. Most, however, are diagnosed on postmortem. The decision to operate is based on the acute onset of weakness, hematochezia, and cardiovascular collapse in conjunction with abdominal radiographs suggestive of a complete obstruction.

Treatment

Rapid surgical intervention is necessary to have any hope for a cure. Because of the severity, signs most often correlate with intestinal ischemia. Intestinal viability cannot be fully evaluated unless the volvulus is reduced (untwisted) and the venous and lymphatic compression is relieved. The inherent dangers of releasing sequestered endotoxins are present when the volvulus is reduced. If tissue necrosis is already present, the involved segment of bowel should be resected without reduction being performed. Crushing clamps are placed at the corners of the volvulus and the mesenteric vasculature is identified, ligated, and divided before removing the twisted segment of bowel. End-to-end anastomosis is then completed as previously described. Euthanasia may be a consideration if the length of the intestine resected exceeds that sufficient to support life. Postoperative care is similar to that described under foreign bodies and intussusseptions.

INTESTINAL INCARCERATION

Incidence/Clinical Signs

The small intestine may translocate, become incarcerated, and ultimately strangulate due to a variety of causes. Diaphragmatic, umbilical, inguinal, femoral, or ventral traumatic hernias and mesenteric rents have all been associated with incarcerations and clinical signs associated with acute intestinal obstruction. Signs of obstruction often closely follow a traumatic incident but occasionally occur spontaneously, after incarceration of the bowel into a hernia of congenital origin. Small diameter tears or rents in the diaphragm, mesentery, or abdominal musculature are more likely to incarcerate and strangulate a segment of intestine than are large defects that often allow to and fro movement of the viscera within the hernia.

The onset of signs will usually be acute and mimic those seen with complete mechanical obstruction. Patients often present with vomiting and progressive dehydration associated with the initial mechanical obstruction. Increased intra-abdominal pressure associated with vomiting or defecation may force the intestine further into the hernial ring. Venous and lymphatic occlusion occurs, leading to congestion and edema of the incarcerated segment. Arterial occlusion and thrombosis can ultimately lead to strangulation and associated signs. Progressive depression, dehydration, electrolyte imbalance, the onset of endotoxic shock, and death may follow.

Diagnosis

The diagnosis of intestinal incarceration with external hernias can often be made on physical exam. Patients showing signs of intestinal obstruction with inguinal, umbilical, femoral, or ventral hernias should be strongly suspected of having an incarcerated intestine. Extreme pain on palpation, with swelling of the hernial area, are distinguishing factors in these cases. Abdominal radiographs may demonstrate dilated gas-filled loops of bowel that end proximal to the hernial ring. Occasionally, gas-filled dilated loops of bowel are seen extra-abdominally in the hernia. With diaphragmatic hernias, a single distended loop of bowel may be noted in the pleural cavity. Occasionally a rent is located dorsally along the diaphragmatic crura, making visualization of the incarceration difficult. A barium sulfate swallow may be necessary to outline the translocated bowel in these cases. Incarceration through a mesenteric rent is usually associated with a prior history of intra-abdominal procedures. Gas- or fluid-filled loops of bowel may be palpated or seen radiographically.

Treatment

Surgical management of incarcerations involves the exposure of the hernia and reduction of the hernial contents, assessment of vascular damage, resection and anastomosis of all devitalized tissue, and, finally, herniorraphy.

With ventral, femoral, or inguinal hernial incarcerations, the skin incision may be located directly over the hernia. However, in most cases it is preferable to make a ventral midline approach. This allows the surgeon to explore the abdominal cavity for additional trauma and to perform the herniorraphy from the peritoneal surface without risk of incorporating underlying structures. Regardless of the approach, relief of the incarceration is facilitated first by enlarging the hernial ring with Metzenbaum scissors. Once the vascular constriction is relieved, the bowel is assessed for its viability. Resection and anastomosis can be performed through the hernial ring, if necessary. However, it is usually best to carefully replace the involved segment of intestine into the abdominal cavity and then to exteriorize it through the midline incision. This allows a better assessment of intestinal viability and easier occlusion of the bowel by the assistant, with less chance for spillage. After relief of the incarceration, the abdominal wall defect is repaired with simple interrupted or mattress sutures of 2-0 to 3-0 nonabsorbable nylon, polypropylene, or stainless steel suture. Mesenteric rents can be closed with a simple continuous pattern of chromic gut, taking care not to include mesenteric vessels in the suture line. Postoperative care is similar to those described under previous sections.

GASTROINTESTINAL PERFORATIONS

Incidence/Clinical Signs

Nontraumatic gastrointestinal perforations may result from gastrointestinal ulcers, sharp penetrating foreign bodies, string foreign bodies, or secondary to necrosis from a mechanical obstruction or incarceration.

The principal sites of peptic ulceration in the dog are the nonacid-producing sites that include the proximal dudodenum, pyloric antrum, and gastric fundus.[1] Perforating gastric ulceration has been reported but is rare in the cat.[22] Ulcers in the dog are almost always associated with an underlying systemic disease process or are drug induced. Bile duct obstruction, mast cell tumors, liver disease, or gastrin-like secreting tumors of the pancreas (Zollinger–Ellison syndrome) have been incriminated. Ulcers have also been associated with oral nonsteroidal anti-inflammatory drugs such as aspirin and phenylbutazone. Gastric and colonic ulcers are reported with greater frequency in dogs with intervertebral disc herniation that have been treated with injectable dexamethazone.[57] Identification of the etiology in ulcer formation is paramount to successful management of the disease. Recent development of H_2-blocking agents such as cimetidine (6–10 mg/kg TID or QID) inhibit histamine-stimulated gastric acid secretion. Sucralfate, another more recent drug used to treat ulcers, binds tightly to the ulcerated mucosa and has numerous properties that enhance the ulcer healing process.

Ulcers can be solitary or multiple. Mucosal erosion precedes ulceration. Common clinical signs include inappetance, intermittent vomiting, melena, regenerative anemia, and abdominal pain. With ulcer perforation, acute abdominal pain, pneumoperitoneum, sudden collapse, and death are common sequelae. A perforation from an ingested foreign body can create signs that range from a localized peritonitis to those associated with generalized peritonitis. Fever, a painful and distended abdomen, and progressive onset of endotoxic shock may be seen. Occasionally, omentum or adjacent mesentery will seal the perforation, and clinical signs will resolve spontaneously.

Diagnosis

The diagnosis of gastrointestinal perforation is usually made radiographically by the presence of free peritoneal air. A fine, radiolucent line may be seen separating the tissue densities of the liver from the diaphragm. If the diagnosis is in question, diagnostic peritoneal lavage may show free bacteria, degenerated WBCs or fecal material. Barium sulfate should be avoided for fear of causing a barium-induced peritonitis. With gastric or proximal duodenal ulcers, the ulceration can often be delineated with a fiberoptic endoscope.

Surgical Repair

When performing an exploratory coeliotomy, complete systematic evaluation of the entire intestinal tract is performed to locate any and all sites of perforation. Small perforations less than .5 mm are debrided back to healthy bleeding tissue and closed with a simple interrupted appositional Gambee or inverting Lembert suture pattern. The surgical site is covered with an omental wrap to act as a seal. If the defect is greater than 5 mm, resection may be necessary or a serosal patch procedure can be performed.

Peptic ulcerations in the gastric fundus may mandate a partial gastrectomy. Peptic ulcerations of the proximal duodenum are often difficult surgical tasks because of their close proximity to the pancreatic duct or common bile duct and major duodenal papilla. If the ulcers are located on the antimesenteric border, they can be debrided and closed or buttressed with a serosal patch or jejunal onlay graft. More commonly, they are located on the mesenteric border. The margins of the ulcer may involve or be closely adjacent to the major duodenal papilla and common bile duct. Resection of the involved proximal duodenum and pylorus is sometimes necessary, and a gastroduodenostomy (Billroth I) or gastrojejunostomy (Billroth II) is performed. If the major duodenal papilla or bile duct is included in the resection, then transposition of the bile duct (choledochoduodenostomy) or gallbladder (cholecystoduodenostomy) must be performed.

SEROSAL PATCHING AND JEJUNAL ONLAY GRAFTING

Indications

Serosal patching utilizes the antimesenteric surface of the small bowel to cover or buttress an adjacent area of questionable tissue viability or an area that cannot be reliably sutured. Jejunum is commonly used because its freely movable mesentery allows it to be mobile. The serosal patch provides mechanical stability and will help to induce and localize a fibrin seal over the questionable area. Serosal patching and jejunal onlay grafting can be used therapeutically to successfully seal intestinal perforations or defects from ulcers, foreign bodies, gun shots, or intestinal dehiscence.[12] It also may be used prophylactically to buttress any hollow organ closure of the stomach, small bowel, colon, urinary bladder, uterus, pancreatic stump, or diaphragm.

Surgical Technique for Serosal Patch

A section of jejunum free of mesenteric tension is transposed over the perforation or area to be buttressed. It is important not to stretch, kink, or twist its mesenteric root, so that the vascular supply will not be disrupted. The bowel chosen for the patch is gently looped to prevent compromise of the lumen. Multiple preforations sometimes require patching using a back-and-forth looping of the entire segment of bowel. The lateral aspect of the bowel wall or antimesenteric border is used for the patch. The patch is not sutured directly to the edges of the defect but rather 3–4 mm beyond its margins. Simple interrupted sutures of 4-0 nylon or polypropylene are placed 3–4 mm from the wound edges and 3–4 mm apart. The sutures grasp the submucosa of the patch and tissue being repaired but do not penetrate the lumen.

Technique for Jejunal Onlay Grafting

The jejunal onlay graft is useful for cases in which a large antimesenteric defect is present in an area where resection or anastomosis is difficult. If the mesenteric border of the duodenum, including the common bile duct, pancreatic duct, or pancreas is preserved, a jejunal onlay pedicle graft can be substituted for complete or partial pancreaticoduodenectomy. An appropriate segment of jejunum is isolated and resected with its mesenteric blood supply intact. Anastomosis of the jejunal segments is then performed. The isolated pedicle graft is incised along its antimesenteric border and then transposed to the donor site without twisting the vasculature. The mucosal surface of the graft is then onlayed over the antimesenteric defect, and the wound edges are apposed with simple interrupted sutures. The jejunal onlay graft has several advantages over the previously described serosal patch. It can be used to cover larger defects, and healthy mucosa faces the lumen of the bowel. The need for mucosal migration over the serosal surface (which occurs with serosal patches) is eliminated.

Management of Peritonitis

Following the reparative surgical procedure, great care is taken to remove all foreign debris, fibrin tags, and devitalized omentum. The abdominal cavity is lavaged with copious amounts of 40°C 0.9 percent NaCl prior to closure. This irrigation is critical in reducing free hemoglobin, vasoactive substances, and bacterial numbers. The use of heparin is advocated by some to diminish adhesion formation. Intra-abdominal placement of antibiotics or povidone-iodine is not recommended. Effective serum levels of parenteral antibiotic therapy can be reached. Since coliform bacteria are likely to be present, antibiotics effective against gram-negative organisms are chosen. Gentamicin–ampicillin combination or trimethoprim–sulfamethoxazole are acceptable for their broad-spectrum bacteriocidal activity. Povidone-iodine lavage of the peritoneal cavity is not recommended because the povidone portion causes renal hypotension in dogs and has produced an increase in the mortality rate of dogs with peritonitis.[32]

SPLENIC NEOPLASIA

Incidence/Clinical Signs

Hemangiosarcoma (HSA) and hemangioma are the most common conditions necessitating splenectomy in the dog.[7] The tumors occur in older dogs with a mean age of 8–10 years. Hemangiosarcoma may be a primary tumor of the spleen or a secondary lesion as a result of metastasis from the right atrium.[19] Surgery may be lifesaving but must be considered palliative since microscopic metastases are usually present at the time of diagnosis. Longevity with splenic hemangiosarcoma is about 6 months, and no known chemotherapy or immunotherapy significantly increases this time.[34] Other primary splenic tumors include fibrosarcoma, lymphosarcoma, plasma cell sarcoma, reticulum cell sarcoma, and mastocytoma. Systemic mastocytosis is the most common indication for splenectomy in the cat and may result in prolonged remission of the disease.[34] These latter tumors do not usually lead to the acute hemorrhagic collapse syndrome seen with splenic HSA and, therefore, will not be within the scope of this chapter.

Clinical signs early in the course include inappetance, periodic vomiting, and weight loss. The latter sign may be due to mechanical displacement of the viscera by the enlarged spleen or merely secondary to cancer cachexia. With advanced tumor growth, blood is lost into the cavernous spaces of the tumor or into the peritoneal cavity from its ulcerative surface. Progressive anemia, weakness, depression, and pale mucous membranes in the presence of a fluid-distended abdomen are suggestive of bleeding hemangiosarcoma. As hemoperitoneum progresses, episodes of syncope or sudden vascular collapse often occur, resulting in a medical and surgical emergency.

Diagnosis

Moderate to severe regenerative anemia is often present with prominent polychromasia and reticulocytosis. A distinguishing feature of HAS in the dog is the presence of nucleated red blood cells in the peripheral blood, with as many as 20/HPF being characteristic.[34] With severe anemia there may be a functional mitral murmur secondary to reduced blood viscosity. Conversely, muffled heart sounds may indicate cardiac tamponade secondary to a lesion in the right auricle. Abdominal paracentesis usually reveals frank venous blood with a packed cell volume similar to that seen peripherally. Neoplastic cells are sometimes identified within the centrifuged buffy coat. Serum liver enzymes (SGPT, SGOT, or SAP) may be increased if hepatic metastasis has occurred.

The splenic mass is usually palpable and identifiable radiographically. In typical cases, a well-defined variably sized spherical mass is seen caudal to the liver shadow. Occasionally, the tail of the spleen is seen adjacent to the mass. Extensive intra-abdominal hemorrhage may obscure visceral outlines. Thoracic radiographs are taken to rule out pulmonary metastasis or hemopericardium secondary to a bleeding right atrium. Needle aspirates of the mass often disclose only frank blood recovered from one of the many cavernous lesions. Definitive diagnosis must be made histologically.

Treatment

As with splenic torsion, preoperative management of hypotension, metabolic acidosis, anemia, ventricular dysrhythmias, and disseminated intravascular coagulation is essential for a successful outcome.

Definitive therapy for splenic hemangiosarcoma involves complete splenectomy. Partial splenectomy is only considered as a diagnostic procedure if the diagnosis is in question. Conditions that may be mistaken for neoplasia include (1) siderotic plaques, which are iron and calcium deposits in the splenic capsule of older animals; (2) benign nodular hyperplasia, which appears as raised symmetrical nodules; (3) large subcapsular hematomas; and (4) splenomegaly. The latter may be drug-induced (by phenothiazine and thiobarbiturates) or secondary to gastric volvulus.

Surgical Technique for Splenectomy

The splenic artery arises from the celiac, sends off branches to the left lobe of the pancreas, and divides into dorsal and ventral branches several centimeters from the spleen. The ventral branch arborizes with the left gastroepiploic artery after supplying the main body of the spleen. The dorsal branch gives rise to the short gastric arteries, after supplying the dorsal extremity of the spleen. Venous drainage is via the splenic vein, which drains into the portal vein via the gastrosplenic vein.

Splenectomy is performed using a ventral midline approach, although extension into a paracostal incision is sometimes needed for large masses. The spleen and the associated mass is gently handled due to its friability and tendency for rupture. Careful inspection of the liver and the remaining abdominal viscera is made for the presence of metastasis. The hilar vessels are isolated, doubly ligated with 2-0 silk, and divided as close to the spleen as possible. The collateral circulation to the stomach is adequate to allow sacrifice of the gastroepiploic and short gastric vessels, if necessary. Mass ligation of the splenic pedicle proximal to the bifurcation of the splenic artery is contraindicated, as ischemia and avascular necrosis of the left pancreatic lobe may result. Following removal of the tumor mass, the abdomen is gently lavaged with warm saline, and the splenic pedicle is examined again for any residual hemorrhage. The splenic lymph nodes are evaluated for evidence of metastasis. Drains are not recommended unless the pancreas or its blood supply have been damaged. Postoperative care and complications are discussed in the following sections.

SPLENIC TORSION

Incidence/Clinical Signs

Splenic torsion or torsion of the splenic pedicle is most commonly seen in 3–6-year-old large deep chested dogs, with the Great Dane at apparent increased risk.[7] Males are possibly predisposed, 6 of 7 cases being males in one study.[56] The condition is frequently seen in association with gastric dilatation-volvulus, but isolated torsion of the spleen alone is well-documented.[56] The exact biomechanics of the torsion have not been elucidated.

Clinical signs vary, some dogs demonstrating acute splenic pain (splenodynia), splenomegaly, cardiovascular collapse, and death within 24 to 48 hours.[41] In other instances, the disease takes a chronic course with anorexia, vomiting, escalating mature neutrophilia, progressive anemia, hemoglobinemia/hemoglobinuria, and eventual progression to shock.[7,40]

Pathophysiology

Splenic torsion results in an acute venous obstruction without arterial occlusion. Large amounts of blood become sequestered in the spleen, and hemolysis is greatly accelerated. Mechanical fragmentation of the cells by intraluminal fibrin stands is the most plausible explanation for this hemolysis.[40] The free hemoglobin and myoglobin may lead to accelerated degenerative changes in the renal tubules, resulting in increased cast production and polyuria. Eventually, splenic arterial thrombosis, widespread splenic infarction and necrosis may result. This favors proliferation of anaerobic organisms and gas production by organisms such as *Clostridia perfringens*, which is a regular contaminant of the canine spleen.[65] Elevations in serum alkaline phosphatase levels are also seen after splenic infarction, both experimentally and clinically.[28,55]

Diagnosis

Splenodynia detected by abdominal palpation or postural gait change is a common finding. Splenomegaly or a mid-abdominal mass is usually detected on palpation and confirmed by abdominal radiographs, although there are no pathognomonic radiographic signs to distinguish torsion from other causes of splenomegaly.

Pallor of the mucous membrane with associated mild to moderate anemia (PCV = 20–25 percent) is common. Erythrocyte regeneration is minimal, with slight polychromasia, target cells, and Howell-Jolly bodies. Hemoglobinemia and hemoglobinuria is common, and darkening of the urine is often seen.

Definitive diagnosis of splenic torsion is usually made on exploratory coeliotomy. The preoperative differential diagnosis for splenomegaly should include neoplasia, hematoma, nodular hyperplasia, and granulomatous or bacterial splenitis. Abdominal paracentesis may differentiate between splenic torsion and neoplasia. Splenic torsion is often not associated with hemoperitoneum, whereas splenic neoplasia usually is.[7]

Treatment

Therapy for splenic torsion includes intravenous infusion of a crystalloid solution or whole blood if the anemia is severe. An exploratory coeliotomy and splenectomy are performed once the patient is stable. Preoperative conditions associated with splenic torsion include hypotension, anemia, metabolic acidosis, ventricular arrythmias, and disseminated intravascular coagulation (DIC). Ventricular arrhythmias may be corrected with either lidocaine (40 μg/kg/min), procainamide (10 mg/kg per os every 6 hr) or quinidine (10–20 mg/kg per os or IM, TID or QID). Metabolic acidosis and DIC due to vascular stasis, anoxia, or inhibition or reticuloendothelial function can usually be overcome with adequate fluid volume replacement in combination with splenectomy. Co-existing septicemia in the presence of splenic necrosis mandates use of intravenous antibiotic therapy. In general, the prognosis for cases of acute collapse after splenic torsion has been guarded to grave. Cases presenting with a more chronic course have been more favorable.[55]

Surgical Technique

Definitive therapy for splenic torsion involves complete splenectomy via a ventral midline approach. Intrasplenic injection of epinephrine will elicit splenic contraction and reduce splenic mass but is not recommended because of the risk of inducing ventricular fibrillation and releasing toxins that are potentially lethal. Most authors suggest untwisting the pedicle prior to splenectomy, but release of bacteria, toxins and cardiodepressive hydrolases are inherent dangers with this approach. Endotoxic shock and ventricular tachycardia has resulted after splenic derotation prior to splenectomy.[55] To alleviate these dangers, the splenectomy may be performed with the spleen twisted and the vessels double clamped and ligated. The short gastric arteries are often avulsed as a result of the splenic torsion. The hilar vessels are ligated as close to the spleen as possible.

Postoperative Care/Complications

Postoperative hypotension may be noted due to relief of pressure on the mesenteric vessels and pooling of blood in the viscera. Postoperative hemorrhage is also common and may be compounded by coexisting DIC. Fluid volume is maintained with balanced electrolyte solution. Cross matched blood transfusions are given as needed to maintain an adequate packed cell volume.

Complications directly related to the surgery include vascular injury to the left lobe of the pancreas with resultant pancreatitis or abscess formation and vascular injury or necrosis of the gastric fundus.[7] Thrombocytosis is a normal sequela after splenectomy and elevated platelet counts of up to three million can be seen for up to 2 weeks postoperatively. Immunologic impairment is not fully determined in the dog, but blood-borne diseases such as hemobartonellosis and babesiasis are more common in splenectomized dogs.

HEPATOBILIARY SYSTEM

Surgical emergencies of the hepatobiliary system are usually traumatically induced. Transcapsular, subcapsular, central hepatic, or biliary tract lacerations are common. A common sequela to a traumatic incident is the development of an intrahepatic hematoma, cyst, or abscess. These patients may present with acute abdominal signs a significant time postinjury.

Nontraumatic surgical emergencies of the liver include liver abscesses and bleeding from ulcerated hepatocellular or cholangiocellular carcinomas. Nontraumatic emergencies of the biliary tract are caused by biliary obstruction due to cholangitis or cholelithiasis.

Liver Abscesses

Incidence/Clinical Signs/Diagnosis. Hepatic abscesses in the dog or cat are extremely rare.[25] Possible etiologies include bacteria, mycotic agents, or protozoa. The liver harbors a normal resident bacteria population with *Clostridium* sp. being the predominant organism.[10] Possible routes of infection include hematogenous spread, ascent through the biliary tract, extension from adjacent organs, penetration by foreign bodies, or surgical manipulation.[51]

Clinical signs include anorexia, vomiting, fever, and abdominal pain, often without associated icterus. Laboratory tests may demonstrate a leukocytosis due to neutrophilia and an elevated SGPT or serum alkaline phosphatase. Both aerobic and anaerobic blood cultures should be examined. Radiographic signs may include lobar enlargement or the presence of gas within the liver parenchyma secondary to gas-forming clostridial organisms.[25] Diagnosis of hepatic abscess is usually made on an exploratory laparotomy or laparoscopy.

Treatment. Treatment for hepatic abscesses involves surgical drainage using Penrose drains or complete excision of the abscess within the offending lobe. Because of the large hepatic reserve, complete removal of the affected lobe is recommended, if possible. Aerobic and anaerobic cultures are taken from the abscess cavity. Because clostridial organisms are always suspected, one of the penicillin-derivative antibiotics are administered intravenously, unless results of bacterial culture and sensitivity dictate otherwise.

Hepatic Neoplasia

Incidence/Clinical Signs. The liver may be involved in both primary and metastatic neoplasms. The order of frequency of primary tumors is hepatocellular carcinoma, hepatoma, cholangiocarcinoma, fibroma/fibrosarcoma, hemangioma/hemangiosarcoma, and hemartomas.[25] Clinical signs include anorexia, vomiting, polyuria, polydypsia, and hepatomegaly. If ulceration and hemorrhage have occurred, progressive anemia, pale mucous membranes, and hemoperitoneum may necessitate emergency surgical intervention.

Prognosis varies with the tumor type. Hepatomas and hepatocellular carcinomas may grow slowly and be confined to single liver lobes, making surgical excision feasible. Cholangiocarcinomas are often associated with weight loss and clinical jaundice. More than one lobe is often affected, and some cases become inoperable. Death usually results within a few months of diagnosis with cholangiocarcinomas.

Diagnosis. Serum chemistries may show profound changes. With hepatocellular carcinoma, SGPT and serum alkaline phosphatase may be increased 10–20-fold.[25] Hypoalbuminemia (less than 2.0 g/dl), hypergamma-globulinemia, hypoglycemia, and hyperbilirubinemia are also commonly noted. Diagnosis of hepatic neoplasia is suspected, based upon palpation and the radiographic presence of a cranial abdominal mass. Displacement of the axis of the stomach caudally is commonly seen. Occasionally the mass may be superimposed over the spleen, making differentiation between splenic and hepatic neoplasms difficult.

Technique for Liver Lobectomy.[6] Five liver lobes are described in the cat and six in the dog. The caudate and right lateral lobes are located to the right of the midline. The right medial and quadrate lobes are midline in location and the left medial and left lateral are to the left of the midline. The blood supply is via the hepatic arteries and portal vein, and venous drainage is through the hepatic veins. Surgical exposure of the liver is accomplished through a ventral midline incision. Anterior extension into a median sternotomy or lateral extension into a left or right paracostal incision is sometimes necessary to gain proper exposure.

Neoplasia, focal abscess formation, or cysts may require partial or total amputation of the affected lobe. Partial hepatectomy may be performed by means of the finger fracture technique. Glisson's capsule and the liver parenchyma are gently compressed between the thumb and middle finger, exposing the hepatic blood vessels and biliary ducts. These are individually ligated with 3-0 chromic catgut or hemoclips, allowing removal of the diseased tissue. If hemorrhage is not adequately controlled, a series of snug mattress sutures are placed through the liver capsule with 2-0 chromic catgut.

Complete lobectomy is performed by careful and tedious isolation of the lobar hepatic artery, vein, and bile duct, respectively. To avoid uncontrollable hemorrhage, the portal vein and hepatic artery can be temporarily occluded. Umbilical tapes are placed around the vessels and passed through the rubber tubing. These are used as tourniquets to occlude the hepatic blood supply if bleeding comes uncontrollable.

A TA55 or TA90 autostapler* may also be used to perform the lobectomy. The instrument is placed across the hepatic pedicle, and a double row of inverted staples occludes the vein, artery, and lobar bile duct, along with adjacent parenchyma. I have noted superior hemostasis and decreased operating time using this technique.

---

* United States Surgical Corporation, Norwalk, CT.

Biliary Tract Obstruction

Incidence/Clinical Signs.   Biliary obstruction may be caused by biliary concretions, stenosis of the common bile duct, neoplasia, cholelithiasis, or choledocholithiasis.[10] Cholelithiasis occurs uncommonly in the dog and even less frequently in the cat.[25] Proposed etiologies for cholelithiasis are bile stasis, infection, changes in bile composition, injury to the bile duct mucosa, and reflux of pancreatic juices. Cholelithiasis does not usually cause overt clinical signs in dogs or cats. Occasionally, choleliths formed in the gallbladder or bile ducts will pass into the common bile duct and cause permanent or temporary obstruction. Bile peritonitis may also result if the cholelith erodes the gallbladder wall.[51] Clinical signs of biliary obstruction include anorexia, vomiting, abdominal pain, and icterus.

Diagnosis.   Evidence of extrahepatic biliary obstruction is suspected with grossly elevated serum bilirubin levels of which 60–90 percent is in the conjugated form.[25] Elevation of urine bilirubin to a 2–3$^+$ level, and absence or reduction of urine urobilinogen levels further substantiates the obstruction. Clinical steatorrhea may also be seen.

Radiographic diagnosis of biliary obstruction is sometimes difficult because only 20–30 percent of the choleliths are radiodense, and oral or intravenous cholecystography is not always successful in identifying gallbladder pathology.[51] The technique of percutaneous cholecystography has been recently described and will distinguish hepatic from posthepatic jaundice. The disadvantage of this technique is that it must be performed under fluoroscopy.[66]

Fluid distention of the abdomen with the recovery of Ictotest positive coffee-colored fluid indicates that bile peritonitis is present and leakage from the hepatobiliary tree has occurred. Exploratory coeliotomy is warranted.

Treatment.   Biliary obstruction should initially be managed by cholecystotomy and exploration of the extrahepatic biliary tree with a probe or catheter. Obstructing calcium bilirubinate stones or inspissated bile may be removed from the gallbladder or dislodged from the bile ducts with saline under pressure. If severe cholangitis or erosion of the gallbladder wall is present, a cholecystectomy should be performed. A cholecystoenterostomy procedure is performed if the calculus can not be dislodged or secondary stricture of the common bile duct is present.

Cholecystotomy.   The gallbladder of the dog and cat is a pear-shaped structure that lies between the quadrate liver lobe medially and the right medial lobe laterally. It is connected to the common bile duct by a single cystic duct. The common bile duct has three or four hepatic lobar ducts that enter at its proximal origin. It then enters the wall of the duodenum obliquely, expands into a well-defined ampulla, and opens into the lumen adjacent to the minor pancreatic duct at the major duodenal papilla.

Stay sutures are initially placed in the fundic region, following isolation and packing off of the gallbladder. Bile is aspirated with a 22-gauge needle and 20 cc syringe to reduce distention before the lumen is entered with a blade. Care is taken to minimize any bile spillage. The contents of the gallbladder are aspirated and all inspissated bile is removed using curettage, saline irrigation, and suction. A 3.5 French infant feeding tube is used to explore and flush the cystic duct, hepatic lobar ducts, and common bile duct to determine patency. If there is increased resistance to flow without apparent extra-hepatic biliary obstruction, potential obstruction at the papilla must be considered, and an enterotomy is performed. Once the obstruction is relieved, the gallbladder is lavaged and closed with a two-layer pattern. A simple continuous layer of 4-0 chromic catgut is covered by a continuous Connell suture pattern using the same suture. The gallbladder is distended with saline solution using a 22-gauge needle and inspected for leakage prior to abdominal closure.

Cholecystectomy. If chronic inflammation or erosion of the gallbladder wall is apparent, cholecystectomy is opted. After cholecystectomy, dilatation of the extrahepatic bile ducts occurs, but detrimental clinical signs have not been noted.[35]

Cholecystectomy can be performed through a transdiaphragmatic incision after performing a right 8th intercostal thoracotomy or through a ventral mid-line/paracostal abdominal approach. After placing a stay suture in the apex of the gallbladder, it is gently dissected from its fossa. Saline may be injected subserosally to identify a better plane between the gallbladder and liver. The cystic artery is identified and ligated. The cystic duct is double-clamped and severed 5 mm from its junction with the common bile duct. The gallbladder is then removed. The abdomen is copiously irrigated before closure.

Cholecystoenterostomy. Bile stasis caused by cholelithiasis, fibrosis with stricture, and invasion of the common bile duct by neoplasia are all reasons why the common bile duct must be bypassed. The small diameter of the canine and feline common bile duct make resection and anastomosis or reimplantation difficult. Side-to-side anastomosis of the gallbladder lumen to the duodenum or jejunum allows retrograde flow of bile away from the obstruction and into the intestinal lumen.

The gallbladder fundus is partially dissected and freed to provide some mobility. The serosa of the jejunum or duodenum is approximated to the gall-bladder serosa for a distance of 3 cm with 4-0 simple interrupted nylon sutures. Two longitudinal 2.5 cm incisions are made in the gallbladder and duodenum closely adjacent to the initial sutures. The mucosal surfaces of the gallbladder and duodenum are then approximated with a continuous Connell suture pattern of 4-0 chromic catgut, thereby creating a stoma. The remaining serosal surfaces are then approximated with simple interrupted 4-0 nylon sutures to prevent bile leakage.

Postoperative Care/Complications. If bile or bacterial peritonitis is present, multiple thorough irrigations of the peritoneal cavity are performed. A sump type of peritoneal catheter may be placed in the vicinity of the gallbladder fossa, and the area may be lavaged with sterile saline for 2–4 days postoperatively. Parenteral antibiotics with a broad spectrum of bacteriocidal activity are given for 7–10 days postoperatively. Adequate hydration is maintained with intravenous crystalloid solution. Postoperative hypoalbuminemia (less than 3 g/percent) may result from effusion of protein from the peritoneal surface.

Whole blood or plasma transfusions may be needed to counteract this loss. Patients are kept NPO for 48 hours postoperatively and then begun on multiple feedings of a low fat ration to diminish cholecystokinin-induced bile secretion.[53]

Ascending cholecystitis has been reported as a common sequela to a cholecystoenterostomy. The pathogenesis is thought to be due to a reflux of duodenal contents into the gallbladder. Clinical signs include fever, abdominal pain, vomiting, neutrophilia, and elevation of SGPT and SGOT.[56] Patients usually respond to oral antibiotic therapy, but recurrent episodes are common. Creation of a stoma at least 2.5 cm in length may decrease gallbladder retention of ingesta and minimize the occurrence of postoperative cholecystitis.[56]

UROGENITAL SYSTEM

Testicular Torsion

Incidence/Clinical Signs. Although testicular torsion is uncommon in dogs, when present, it may require immediate surgical attention. The condition occurs almost exclusively in cryptorchid animals, and in unilateral cryptorchids the torsion invariably involves the retained abdominal testicle.[46] Intrascrotal testicular torsion has been described but is less common than intra-abdominal torsion. The degree of intra-abdominal spermatic cord torsion varies between 180° and 900°, and there appears to be an equal incidence on the left and right sides.[41,47]

Testicular torsion can occur in young dogs less than a year of age without evidence of preexisting testicular disease or in older, mature dogs (3–10 years) in which there is a 70 percent incidence of neoplasia.[41] The most common neoplasm associated with testicular torsion is Sertoli cell tumor, seminoma and interstitial cell tumors being much less common.[41]

Most patients with torsion of an intra-abdominal testicle present with an acute onset of abdominal pain. Clinical signs include splinted abdomen, tenesmus, anorexia, and vomiting. A painful enlarged caudal abdominal mass is sometimes palpated caudal to the kidneys. Dehydration may be present in cases with protracted emesis. With torsion of an intrascrotal testicle, there is usually an acute onset of scrotal pain and edema, with rear limb stiffness.[47]

The etiology of intra-abdominal testicular torsion is unknown, but the proposed hypotheses include fixation of the testicle by peritoneal bands, rotation around a fixed point caused by bowel movement, an abnormally long gubernaculum, spasm of the cremaster muscle, and increased weight and mobility of the testicle secondary to neoplasia.[41] Enlargement of the rotated testicle may be due to venous occlusion with resultant inflammation and edema or may be secondary to neoplasia.

Diagnosis. Testicular torsion is suspected upon palpation of a painful mid- to caudal abdominal mass in a cryptorchid animal. The mass is sometimes visible on abdominal radiographs. Differential diagnoses include prostatic abscess, localized peritonitis, and intestinal obstruction. Definitive diagnosis is usually only possible on exploratory coeliotomy.

Treatment. Management of testicular torsion involves an exploratory coeliotomy and orchiectomy. Fluid and electrolyte imbalances are corrected preoperatively. A ventral midline incision is made via a parapreputial skin incision. The testicle is usually 2–3 times normal size and is engorged with blood. The ductus deferens and spermatic vessels are isolated and doubly ligated with 2-0 chromic catgut. If testicular necrosis is evident, ligation and division of the spermatic cord is made prior to untwisting of the testicle. The specimen is submitted to histopathology in an attempt to document neoplasia. If the opposite testicle is retained, it is removed at this time.

Prophylactic antibiotics are given during surgery and for 48–96 hours postoperatively, if testicular necrosis or an abscess is present. Residual fluid and electrolyte imbalances are managed postoperatively. Prognosis is good in uncomplicated cases.

Prostatic Abscesses

Most nontraumatic diseases of the prostate do not require emergency surgery. However, prostatic abscesses or infected prostatic cysts may become extremely large and go unnoticed before rupturing and causing severe localized peritonitis. An acute abdominal crisis often ensues which requires immediate surgical attention.

Incidence/Clinical Signs. Suppurative prostatitis usually occurs secondarily to benign prostatic hyperplasia and is often seen in dogs greater than 5 years of age. No particular breed predeliction is reported. Common bacterial agents include *Proteus, Pseudomonas, E. coli, Staphylococcus* and Streptococcus sp. A history of tenesmus, stranguria, and hematuria or pyuria (at the end of urination) is often reported. After urination, the animal often remains in a squatting posture and may strain for several seconds before blood is seen.

The prostate is usually dropped over the pelvic brim and often pushes the urinary bladder rostrally. Manipulating the gland into the pelvic canal by abdominal palpation sometimes makes rectal palpation possible. The gland is often firm and assymetrical, but the abscess center may feel smooth and fluctuant. Depression, fever, anorexia, vomiting and posterior abdominal splinting are usually noted with abscess rupture. Bacterial peritonitis may progress to endotoxic shock, progressive cardiovascular collapse, and death.

Diagnosis. Varying degrees of hematuria, pyuria, and bacteriura may be seen on urinalysis. Bacterial cystitis is usually present concurrently, and recent evidence indicates that a prostatic ejaculate appears to be the most dependable source for bacterial isolation.[23] A marked elevation of the peripheral white cell count is usually not seen in the uncomplicated abscesses with counts of 9–17,000 common in one report.[30] If the abscess ruptures, secondary peritonitis results, and neutrophilia with the presence of immature cells is commonly seen.[30]

Plain film radiography usually reveals an enlarged mass at the pelvic brim or posterior abdominal cavity with dorsal displacement of the colon. Occasionally a large paraprostatic abscess will be located in the pelvic canal or anterior to the bladder. Positive contrast retrograde cysturethrography will delineate bladder location. Reflux of dye from the prostatic urethra into the glandular parenchyma may occur but does not necessarily distinguish a suppurative prostatitis from other types of prostatic disease. Radiographs do not distinguish between prostatic abscesses and cysts. Other signs, including fever, glandular pain, pyuria, and evidence of localized peritonitis provide enough anecdotal information to give a presumptive diagnosis of prostatic abscess. Abdominocentesis or diagnostic peritoneal lavage may indicate degenerated PMNs and the presence of intracellular bacteria. A single bacterial species is usually seen with a prostatic abscess, whereas in gastrointestinal leakage, a positive lavage will often reveal multiple bacterial species. Percutaneous needle biopsy of the gland is not recommended because of the danger of rupturing a large abscess.

Treatment.   Conservative management of uncomplicated prostatic abscesses is usually unrewarding. Ruptured abscesses are frequently associated with a high degree of mortality. Regardless of the surgical technique used, castration is performed as an ancillary procedure in all cases, in order to facilitate glandular atrophy. Fluid and electrolyte replacement therapy is performed prior to surgery, is possible. If abscess rupture has occurred and in spite of aggressive therapy the patient cannot be stailized, a coeliotomy is performed as rapidly as possible.

Gross pathologic changes seen with prostatic abscesses vary greatly. The gland may be diffusely involved, with multiloculated small compartments, or the abscess pockets may coalesce to form one or more large abscesses (Fig. 8-4). The abscess cavity may or may not communicate with the urethra. A distinguishing factor of large, single-compartment abscesses is the thick, indurated capsule which often differs from the thin, fibrous capsule seen with prostatic cysts. Aspiration of the fluid contents usually distinguishes between the two, abscesses having purulent or sanguinopurulent fluid with greater than 10,000 WBCs/mm^2. Cysts usually contain clear or serosanguinous fluid.

Most prostatic abscesses can be managed by marsupialization or ventral tube drainage. Abscesses located in the pelvic canal within a perineal hernia may be drained through the perineum. Total prostatectomy is not indicated for prostatic abscesses, because of the risk of postoperative urinary incontinence or dehiscence of the suture line.

Surgical Technique.   Prostatic surgery is performed through a caudal–ventral midline incision extending from the umbilicus to the pubis. The marsupialization technique is reserved for unruptured, large, single cavity abscesses. The abscess wall must be sutured to the skin with minimal tension, since dehiscence and abdominal leakage may result in fatal peritonitis. A small stab incision is made through the abscess wall; the abscess is then drained by means of suction. Cultures and biopsies are then taken. The abscess wall is exteriorized through a 4–6 cm paramedian incision extending through the skin and abdominal muscles. The abscess wall is sutured to the musculature with 2-0 simple interrupted nylon sutures, incorporating peritoneum and abdominal musculature in the sutures. The stab incision is then enlarged to 3 cm and

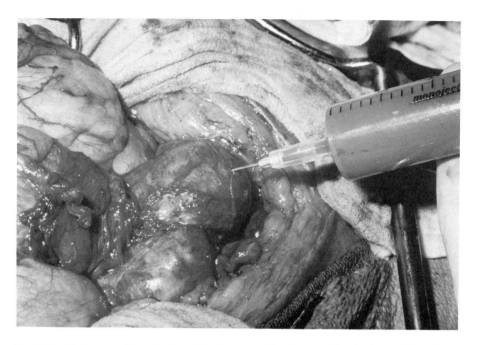

Fig. 8-4. Intraoperative photograph of a prostatic abscess. Aspiration of the abscess reveals purulent exudate. Drainage of these lobes can be accomplished using either Penrose or Foley catheters.

sutured to the skin with 3-0 simple interrupted nylon to complete the stoma. The abdomen is lavaged vigorously and routine closure is performed.

Aftercare consists of daily irrigation of the abscess cavity with saline or povidine-iodine solution. Petrolatum is applied around the marsupialization stoma to reduce skin irritation. Drainage subsides gradually over the first week, but efforts are made to keep the stoma open as long as possible. Daily swabbing of the stoma with a cotton-tipped applicator sometimes will keep it open for 3–4 weeks.

Multiloculated prostatic abscesses and ruptured abscesses are best handled with ventral tube drainage. A stab incision is made into the ventral prostatic capsule, and the abscess is drained. Culture and sensitivity and biopsies are taken at this time. Septa between pus-filled cavities are gently broken down by digital palpation to create a single large cavity. The abscess cavity is then irrigated with sterile saline solution. A separate stab incision is placed in the dorsal capsule, and 2¼-inch Penrose drains are run through the glandular parenchyma from ventral to dorsal and secured to the capsule with simple interrupted 4-0 chromic catgut sutures. They are then exteriorized through stab incisions on both sides of the midline and secured to the skin with 3-0 nylon. Three additional Penrose drains are placed to drain the paraprostatic area on either side of the gland and exit the abdomen in similar fashion. The caudal abdominal cavity is copiously lavaged, and closure of the linea alba is performed with simple interrupted nonabsorable nylon or polypropylene.

In instances where the abscess is well-defined in one or both prostatic lobes, a Foley catheter can be placed through a small stab incision made in the ventral aspect of the lobe, following the placement of a purse-string suture. Two catheters are necessary for bilateral involvement. An instrument or a small finger is placed through the stab wound to break down any septa prior to catheter placement. The bulb portion of the catheter is then inflated, and the ends of the catheter are allowed to exit through stab incisions in the abdominal wall just lateral to the midline abdominal incision. The catheters are flushed daily with saline and remain in place for 7–10 days before being removed.

Postoperative Care/Complications. The dog is fitted with an Elizabethean collar to prevent drain removal. Aggressive parental antibiotic therapy is continued for 7–14 days postoperatively. The choice of antibiotic remains controversial. Most antibiotics are unable to cross the prostatic epithelial barrier in normal dogs. Of the commonly used antibiotics only erythromycin, oleandomycin, and trimethoprim sulfa obtain adequate concentrations in normal prostatic fluid. However, with bacterial prostatitis, the blood/prostatic fluid barrier is broken down. This may explain why penicillins, sulfas, aminoglycosides, and tetracylines have been used to successfully treat bacterial prostatitis. It is therefore recommended that the patient be started on trimethoprim sulfa 15 mg/kg bid postoperatively and if clinical response is not adequate, the choice of antibiotics is changed according to the results of a culture and sensitivity. The drains within the prostatic capsule are pulled out 7–10 days after surgery, depending on the quantity of fluid drainage. The paraprostatic drains are pulled 2 days after the abscess drains are removed.

When there is communication of the abscess cavity with the prostatic urethra or finger dissection has been too aggressive, urine leakage through the drains often occurs.[23] This problem usually resolves spontaneously, although passage of an indwelling urethral catheter may be necessary for 4–5 days.

Toxic Pyometra

Incidence/Clinical Signs. Pyometra may manifest itself as an acute or chronic disease with variable systemic clinical signs. The disease can be loosely divided into an early phase that can be managed on an elective basis and a toxemic phase that becomes a medical and surgical emergency. The disease usually occurs in dogs, 5 years of age or older and within 12 weeks of the last observed estrus.[26] Clinical signs vary depending on the severity of uterine pathology, the presence or abscence of bacteria, the duration of the illness, and the patency of the cervix. Common clinical signs include depression, anorexia, vomiting, polydipsia, polyuria, and vaginal discharge. When the cervix is open, the discharge is often grey or brown and has a fetid odor. Dogs with closed pyometra accumulate large quantities of pus within the uterus, and abdominal enlargement is occasionally seen. These dogs tend to become more depressed and toxic than those with an open cervix.

Diagnosis.   Tentative diagnosis of toxic pyometra is possible in the depressed, prostrate, or markedly dehydrated animal that presents with vaginal discharge and palpable uterine enlargement. Careful palpation is mandatory, because the friable uterus is easily ruptured. The presence of a homogeneous, fluid-filled, tubular structure in the caudal abdomen further confirms the diagnosis. Compression (paddle) techniques may move the intestines out of the way in cases that are difficult to diagnose. Free peritoneal fluid may indicate that the pyometra has ruptured and immediate exploratory coeliotomy is warranted.

Glomerulonephropathy may result from the deposition of immune complexes in glomerular capillary walls, resulting in proteinuria. Polyuria and compensatory polydypsia result from an impaired capacity to concentrate the urine (sp gr < 1.010). Dehydration may develop to a degree sufficient to cause poor renal perfusion, and prerenal azotemia results in anorexia and/or vomiting. Accumulation of neutrophils in the uterus usually causes a marked regenerative left shift. White counts of 30,000 or 100,000 are commonly seen. However, in severely toxic animals a degenerative left shift and nonregenerative anemia may result from bone marrow depression.

Treatment.   Careful attention to fluid and electrolyte deficiencies is necessary to combat shock and to reduce the chance of secondary renal complications commonly associated with toxic pyometra. Adequate hydration is necessary to maintain an acceptable glomerular filtration rate. Continuous infusion of 20 percent mannitol at 0.5–1.0 g/kg before and after surgery may help to prevent acute renal shutdown. Broad-spectrum bacteriocidal antibiotics are administered to counteract preexisting sepsis and the danger of peritoneal contamination during the surgery.

Definitive surgery for toxic pyometra involves ovariohysterectomy. Medical management using transcervical tube drainage and lavage, oxytocin/estrogen combinations, prostaglandin F_2 alpha, and surgical removal of the corpus luteum are reserved for valuable breeding animals with uncomplicated pyometra.

Surgical Techniques.   The choice of anesthesia depends on the degree of toxicity present. The procedure can often be performed in prostrate animals with a local 2 percent lidocaine block and a 1:1 ratio of nitrous oxide and oxygen administered via mask. Mask induction and intubation with halothane and oxygen may also be used.

A standard ovariohysterectomy via a ventral midline incision is performed. Care must be taken not to rupture the friable uterus as it is manipulated out of the abdominal incision. After double ligation of the uterine artery and vein, the uterus is doubly clamped and removed. The uterine contents are aspirated away from the surgical field and submitted for culture. The uterine stump should be shortened to within 5 mm of the cervix. The cut edge is inverted by using a continuous Cushing pattern with 2-0 chromic catgut. The peritoneal cavity is liberally lavaged with warm normal saline solution prior to abdominal closure.

Postoperative Management.   Fluid therapy commensurate with replacement and maintenance needs are continued in the postoperative period. An indwelling urinary catheter can be placed to monitor urinary output. Postoperative parenteral antibiotics are continued for 48 hours. After hysterectomy, the WBC count usually exceeds preoperative levels. The leukocytosis remains for a few days but does not indicate infection. Glomerular lesions are usually reversible, and proteinuria resolves adequately. Likewise, the ability to concentrate urine occurs when normal medullary hypertonicity is restored.[26]

Uterine Torsion

Incidence/Clinical Signs.   Torsion of one or both uterine horns has been reported in the dog and the cat. Ovarian torsion may accompany uterine torsion or it may occur independently, with a neoplastic ovary. Uterine torsion usually occurs in pregnant animals. In one study, 5 of 8 dogs with uterine torsion were gravid bitches, and in the cat 8 of 8 were pregnant queens.[31] Uterine torsion in a nulliparous, nongravid bitch is also reported.[29] The exact etiology is unknown, but uterine tumors, anatomic anomalies, excessive fetal movement, and uterine adhesions have been suggested as possible causes. Uterine torsion usually occurs at the end of pregnancy or during parturition, but it has also been described as early as 6 weeks of gestation. The degree of torsion can vary from 180° to 2,160° (six rotations).[31]

Clinical signs of uterine torsion depend upon the degree of rotation or the amount of ischemia. Rapid onset of dystocia, abdominal pain, and restlessness may be the initial signs. Severe weakness, prolonged capillary profusion, tachycardia, weak pulse, and hypothermia may occur if uterine congestion and ischemia are pronounced. Occasionally, the vascular compromise is minimal and animals with uterine torsion are asymptomatic.

Definitive diagnosis of uterine torsion is usually made during exploratory coeliotomy after other causes of acute abdomen have been ruled out. Palpation of the affected horn is difficult because of the full term pregnancy status of the animal. Rectal or vaginal examination is usually unrewarding. Radiography may indicate a fluid-dense mass in the caudal ventral abdomen.

Treatment.   Definitive management of uterine torsion usually involves ovariohysterectomy, because uterine ischemia is often present at the time of surgery. If unilateral torsion and necrosis have occurred in the valuable breeding animal, hysterectomy of the torsed horn may be followed by hysterotomy and evacuation of fetuses from the unaffected horn.[24] Postoperative management involves supportive fluid and electrolyte therapy. Prophylactic antibiotics are indicated perioperatively if uterine necrosis has occurred.

Urethral Obstruction

Incidence/Clinical Signs.   Obstruction of the urethra by calculi is the most common surgical emergency involving the urinary tract in the dog and cat. Males become obstructed more than females because of the anatomic reduction in the penile urethral diameter. The mean age for urolithiasis is 5.5 years in dogs and 5.8 years in cats.[8,42]

In the dog, male to female ratio is greatly dependent on the calculus type. Phosphate (struvite) calculi are usually seen in conjunction with a cystitis caused by urease-producing bacteria. Adult females are affected more than males, although in immature (less than 1 year old) animals there is a higher incidence of calculi in the male. Urate and oxalate calculi are predominently seen in the male, with silicate and cystine calculi being reported almost exclusively in male dogs.[8]

In the cat, the feline urologic syndrome (FUS) may be caused by urethral plugs seen exclusively in males or uroliths seen in the males and females. Urethral plugs contain varying quantities of proteinaceous material, cellular debris, and magnesium ammonium phosphate (struvite) crystals and are usually not associated with bacterial cystitis. Conversely, uroliths are organized, crystalline aggregates that are usually composed of struvite and are radiodense. Urease-producing bacteria are present in some of these cases.

The dog with cystic calculi or the cat with unobstructed FUS usually demonstrates signs consistent with cystitis. Pollakiuria, stranguria, and hematuria are seen. In the male dog, the calculi often pass along the urethra and lodge at the caudal aspect of the os penis. Single or multiple calculi may lodge at this site, and signs will vary from those indicating partial obstruction (dysuria) to that of complete obstruction (anuria). Similar signs are seen in the cat with partial or complete urethral obstruction. When complete urethral obstruction is present, rapid progression to postrenal azotemia, emesis, dehydration, metabolic acidosis, hyperkalemia, and hypothermia occurs.

Diagnosis.   Diagnosis of complete urethral obstruction is based on clinical signs and palpation of a greatly distended, turgid bladder. Attempts at expressing urine are usually unrewarding, but occasionally a few drops of bloody urine will dribble from the penile urethra. Plain film radiography may indicate the presence of radiopaque cystic or urethral calculi. Contrast retrograde urethrography is often helpful in diagnosing radiolucent urethral calculi in the dog. The penile urethra is best viewed with the legs pulled caudally; the perineal urethra is seen best with the legs pulled rostrally. In the cat, the obstruction is commonly located in the penile urethra near its tip. The tip of the penis is hyperemic, and often the calculi or urethral plug can be palpated by gently rolling the penis between the thumb and index finger.

Treatment.   Treatment for acute urethral obstruction involves relief of the obstruction and supportive medical care. This section will focus on relief of the obstruction and medical management. Detailed descriptions of the many urethrostomy techniques are beyond the scope of this chapter.

Initial management of the patient depends on the acid–base, electrolyte, and hydration status as well as the degree of uremia. Acidemia may be treated using alkalinizing electrolyte solutions such as Multisol* which contains 53 mEq/L $NaHCO_3$. The volume of fluid administered is based on the severity of dehydration. Dehydration is corrected as rapidly as possible to reestablish renal

---

* Abbott Laboratories, North Chicago, IL.

blood flow. A five percent dehydration is mild, 8 percent is moderate, and 12 percent is severe.[2] Fluid deficit replacement is administered over 1–2 hours and should not exceed 50–60 ml/kg/hr in the cat, or pulmonary edema may develop. Although hyperkalemia can be treated with intravenous infusions of dextrose and/or insulin, increased survivability with this technique has not been documented.[52] A more reliable and safer method of treating the hyperkalemia is to restore circulatory volume and increase renal perfusion, which, in turn, increases renal excretion of potassium. In addition, correction of acidemia causes increased cellular uptake of potassium which aids in the reduction of the serum hyperkalemia.

Relief of obstruction in the cat is usually accomplished by retrograde flushing of the penile urethra to remove the urethral plug or calculus. Open-ended polyethylene catheters* or blunt lacrimal cannulas may be used for this purpose. The obstruction can often be relieved without sedation, using lidocaine gel in the moribund animal, or with a low dose of ketamine (2–4 mg/kg IV) in other cases. If a good stream of urine is noted with adequate bladder detrusor function, the urethra is not left catheterized. The urethra and bladder are catheterized with a 3.5 French rubber catheter, if the urethral stream is poor, if urethral trauma is severe, if bladder atony is present, or if renal failure is suspected and urine output must be monitored. Indwelling catheters will increase gross hematuria, due to bladder wall trauma, urethritis, and an increased tendency for postoperative cystitis.[42] If the urethral plug cannot be removed, cystocentesis is performed, followed by a repeated attempt at catheterization. If this is unsuccessful, an emergency perineal urethrostomy may be required. Another alternative may be the placement of a percutaneous, suprapubic, Stamey urinary drainage catheter.† The animal may then be stabilized and a perineal urethrostomy performed on an elective basis. The catheter is a 10 French, polyethlene catheter with 4 wings at the tip and an 18-gauge stylet. It is introduced into the bladder lumen percutaneously after aseptic preparation.[5] When the stylet is removed, the wings of the catheter extend outward, forming a circular configuration at its tip and preventing migration out of the bladder lumen. The catheter is then secured to the skin with a piece of adhesive tape and 3-0 nylon. Removal involves reinsertion of the stylet, which straightens the wings and facilitates catheter removal.

Relief of urethral obstruction in the dog can usually be accomplished nonsurgically under deep sedation or general anesthesia. With 1–3 urethral calculi and no cystic calculi, normograde urohydropropulsion is initially attempted.[48] An 8–12 French rubber or foley catheter is lubricated and inserted 2–3 cm into the urethra. The urethra is dilated by injecting saline under pressure while digitally occluding the external urethral orifice around the catheter and having an assistant simultaneously compressing the pelvic urethra via rectal palpation. When the assistant feels that the urethra has dilated to twice normal size, the

---

* Open End Tom Cat Catheter, Sovereign Labs, St Louis, MO.
† Stamey Suprapubic Catheter, 10 French, Cook Urological, Spencer, IN.

penile urethral catheter is quickly withdrawn while maintaining pelvic urethral pressure. Small calculi may then move past the os penis and out of the urethra, relieving the obstruction. If this method fails, or, if multiple urethral and cystic calculi are present, the calculi can sometimes be flushed back into the bladder with retrograde saline flushes. Occasionally, retrograde urohydropropulsion is needed to relieve the obstruction. With retrograde urohydropropulsion, the urethra is distended as previously described, but the assistant rapidly removes pressure from the pelvic urethra, allowing retrograde movement of saline and calculi into the bladder. The procedure is repeated until the urethra is clear of all calculi. An indwelling catheter may then be retained, allowing patient stabilization and cystotomy on an elective basis. If urohydropropulsion is not successful at dislodging urethral calculi, emergency cystocentesis may be performed, followed by a urethrotomy to remove the calculi or a permanent urethrostomy proximal to the obstruction.

Indications for urethrostomies are: (1) calculi that cannot be removed nonsurgically, (2) strictures caused by previous surgery or chronic calculi lodgement, and (3) prevention of obstruction in dogs with rapidly recurring urolithiasis. In the dog, urethrostomies are performed in the perineal, prepubic, or scrotal locations. The perineal location is not recommended in the dog because of postoperative scrotal urine burns and propensity for hemorrhage and stricture formation. However, perineal urethrostomy may be necessary when obstruction or stricture are located at the ischial arch. The prepubic urethrostomy is made immmediately caudal to the os penis. The advantage of the procedure is that the scrotum and testicles are salvaged. The disadvantages are: (1) the urethra is surrounded by much cavernous tissue and bleeding is often profound, and (2) the urethra is somewhat narrow, and stricture is more likely. Scrotal urethrostomy is the preferred technique by most surgeons because: (1) the urethra is more superficial at this location and contains less cavernous tissue; (2) the urethra is wide so that stones are passed with greater ease; and (3) ventral drainage of urine is good, and skin scalds are rare. The disadvantages of scrotal urethrostomy are that castration and scrotal ablation must be performed.

If cystic calculi are still present after the relief of obstruction, a cystotomy is performed. If the animal is not uremic, the urethrostomy and cystotomy are performed at the same time. If the animal is uremic, urethrostomy is performed to relieve obstruction, and cystotomy is performed at a later date. A specimen for culture and sensitivity is taken from a piece of the bladder mucosa or the interior of the calculus. Some stones should be submitted for crystallography. Multiple passages of the urethral catheter along with saline flushes are necessary to assure removal of all calculi. Closure is performed with a continuous Cushing pattern of 3-0 polygalactin 910.

Postoperative Care/Complications. Fluid therapy is continued postoperatively until azotemia, hyperkalemia, and postoperative diuresis have resolved. Hyperkalemia usually abates within 24 hours, but postoperative obstructive hypokalemia may result and may require supplementation of 20 mEq KCl to each liter of balanced electrolyte solution. Azotemia often falls to within normal limits within 72 hours.

Bladder atony may result from bladder detrusor muscle dysfunction. An indwelling urethral catheter may be required to keep the bladder emptied for several days and to allow tight junctions of the detrusor muscle to reform. Oral bethanacol (2.5 mg TID) can also be used to facilitate bladder emptying. Patency of the urethra must be insured when using this drug, because if residual obstruction is present, rupture of the bladder may occur. Treatment of a concurrent bacterial cystitis is done with appropriate antibiotics as determined by culture and sensitivity. Postoperative dietary management, urine acidification or alkalination, antimetabolite therapy, and antimicrobial management are critical to reducing the recurrence of specific types of canine and feline uroliths. The recent development of prescription medical dietary regimens effecting dissolution of canine struvite uroliths has also been described.[43] Dietary management of aseptic struvite uroliths has been successful in many instances with dissolution of the stones occurring in 8 to 20 weeks.

REFERENCES

1. Ader P: Penetrating gastric ulceration in a dog. J Am Vet Med Assoc 175:710, 1979
2. Barsanti JA, Finco DR: Feline urologic syndrome: medical therapy. p. 1108. In Kirk RW (ed): Current Veterinary Therapy VIII. WB Saunders, Philadelphia, 1983
3. Betts CW, Wingfield WE, Green RW: A retrospective study of gastric dilation-torsion in the dog. J Small Anim Pract 15:727, 1974
4. Bone DL, Duckett KE, Patton CS, Krahwinkel DJ: Evaluation of anastomosis of small intestine in dogs: crushing versus noncrushing suturing techniques. Am J Vet Res 44(11):2043, 1983
5. Botte RJ: Percutaneous prepubic urinary drainage in normal cats. Vet Surg 13(4):202, 1983
6. Breznock EM: Liver, biliary system and pancreas. p. 205. In Bojrab MJ (ed): Current Techniques in Veterinary Surgery II. Lea & Febiger, Philadlephia, 1983
7. Brodey RS: The spleen. p. 818. In Archibald J: Canine Surgery II. 2nd Ed. American Veterinary Publications, Santa Barbara, 1974
8. Brown NW, Parks JC, Green RW: Canine urolithiasis: retrospective analysis of 438 cases. J Am Vet Med Assoc 176:415, 1977
9. Chatworthy HW, Saleeby R, Lovingood C: Extensive small bowel resection in young dogs: its effect on growth and development. Surgery 32(2):341, 1952
10. Cobb LM, McKay KA: A bacteriological study of the liver of the normal dog. J Compar Pathol 72:92, 1962
11. Crowe DT: Diagnostic abdominal paracentesis techniques: clinical evaluation in 129 dogs and cats. J Am Anim Hosp Assoc 20(2):223, 1984
12. Crowe DT: The serosal patch: clinical use in 12 animals. Vet Surg 13(1):29, 1984
13. Dillon AR, Spano JS: The acute abdomen. p. 461. In Dillon AR (ed): Symposium on Gastroenterology: Veterinary Clinics of North America. WB Saunders, Philadelphia, 1983
14. Ellison GW, Volcinen MC, Park RD: End to end intestinal anastomosis in the dog. A comparative fluorescein dye, angiographic and histopathologic evaluation. J Am Anim Hosp Assoc 18(5):729, 1982

15. Ellison GW: End to end intestinal anastomosis in the dog. A comparison of techniques. Comp Cont Ed Small Anim Pract 3(6):486, 1981

16. Engen MK: Bowel plication for preventing recurrent intussusception. p. 113. In Bojrab MJ, (ed): Current Techniques in Small Animal Surgery II. WB Saunders, Philadelphia, 1983

17. Enquist IF, Bauman FG, Rehder E: Changes in body fluid spaces in dogs with intestinal obstruction. Surg Gynecol Obstet 127:17, 1968

18. Fallah AM: Circumcostal gastropexy in the dog: a preliminary study. Vet Surg 11:9, 1982

19. Fees DL, Withrow SJ: Canine hemangiosarcoma. Comp Cont Ed Small Anim Pract 3(12):1049, 1981

20. Funkquist B: Gastric torsion in the dog I: radiological picture during nonsurgical treatment related to the pathological anatomy and to the further clinical course. J Small Anim Pract 20:73, 1979

21. Funkquist B, Obel N: Gastric torsion in the dog II. Nonsurgical treatment by aspiration of gastric contents during repeated rotation of the animal. J Small Anim Pract 20:93, 1979

22. Gordon RN: A perforating gastric ulcer in a cat. Aust Vet J 56:41, 1980

23. Greiner TP, Johnson RG: Diseases of the prostate gland. p. 1459. In Ettinger SJ (ed): Textbook of Veterinary Internal Medicine, II. WB Saunders, Philadelphia, 1983

24. Hall MA, Sevenberg LN, Genital Emergencies. p. 1224. In Kirk, RW (ed): Current Veterinary Therapy VII. WB Saunders, Philadelphia, 1980

25. Hardy RM: Diseases of the liver. p. 1372. In Ettinger SJ (ed): Textbook of Veterinary Internal Medicine. WB Saunders, Philadelphia, 1983

26. Hardy RM, Senior DF: Canine pyometra. p. 1216. In Kirk RW (ed): Current Veterinary Therapy VII. WB Saunders, Philadelphia, 1980

27. Harvey HJ, Rendano VT: Small bowel volvulus in dogs: clinical observations. Vet Surg 13(2):91, 1984

28. Hightman BEC, Thomson J, Roshe J, Altland PD: Serum alkaline phosphatase in dogs with experimental splenic and renal infarcts with endocarditis. Proc Soc Exp Biol Med 95:109, 1957

29. Homer BL, Altman NH: Left uterine torsion in a non-gravid nulliparous bitch. J Am Vet Med Assoc 176(7):633, 1980

30. Hornbuckle WE: Prostatic disease in the dog. Cornell Vet 68(7):284, 1978

31. Johnston SD: Management of pregnancy disorders in the bitch and queen. p. 954. In Kirk RW (ed): Current Veterinary Therapy VIII. WB Saunders, Philadelphia, 1983

32. Lagarde MC, Balton JS: Intraperitoneal povidone-iodine in experimental peritonitis. Ann Surg 186(6):613, 1978

33. Lipowitz AJ: Intestinal obstruction in the dog. California Vet 3(1):8, 1980

34. Liska WD, MacEwan EG, Zaki FA, Garvey M: Feline systemic mastocytosis: a review and results of splenectomy in seven cases. J Am Anim Hosp Assoc 15:589, 1979

35. Mahour GH, Wahin KG, Saule EH, Ferris DO: Effect of cholecystectomy on the biliary ducts in the dog. Arch Surg 97:570, 1968

36. Marks DL: Canine pylorogastric intussusception. Vet Med/Sm Anim Clin 5:677, 1983

37. McCoy DM: A gastropexy technique for permanent fixation of the pyloric antrum. J Am Anim Hosp Assoc 18:763, 1982

38. McLackin AD: Omental protection of intestinal anastomosis. Am J Surg 125:134, 1973

39. Mishra NK, Appert HE, Howard JM: The effects of distension and obstruction on the accumulation of fluid in the lumen of small bowel of dogs. Ann Surg 180:791, 1974

40. Moreau PM, Henley MW: Fatal clostridial splenitis secondary to splenic torsion. Canine Pract 8(3):55, 1981

41. Naylor RW, Thompson SMR: Intraabdominal testicular torsion: a report of two cases. J Am Anim Hosp Assoc 15(6):763, 1979

42. Osborn CA, Johnston GR: Feline urolithiasis. p. 1076. In Kirk RW (ed): Current Veterinary Therapy VIII. WB Saunders, Philadelphia, 1983

43. Osborne CA, Klausner JS, Kraweic DR, Griffith DP: Canine struvite urolithiasis: problems and their dissolution. J Am Vet Med Assoc 179:2239, 1981

44. Parks JC, Greene RW: Tube gastrostomy for the treatment of gastric volvulus. J Am Anim Hosp Assoc 12:168, 1976

45. Pass MA, Johnston DR: Treatment of gastric dilatation-torsion in the dog: gastric decompression by gastrostomy under local analgesia. J Small Anim Pract 14:131, 1973

46. Pearson H: Testicular torsion in the dog: a review of thirteen cases. Vet Rec 97(11):200, 1975

47. Peduzzi RJ, Calson DJ: Testicular torsion. Canine Pract 7(13):79, 1980

48. Piermattei DL, Osborne GA: Nonsurgical removal of calculi from the urethra of a male dog. J Am Vet Med Assoc 159:1755, 1971

49. Randall HT: Fluid, electrolyte and acid–base balance. Surg Clin North Am 56: WB Saunders, Philadelphia, 1976.

50. Reymond RD: The mechanism of intussusception: a theoretical analysis of the phenomenon. Br J Radiol 45:7, 1972

51. Rubin GJ, Jones BT: The liver. p. 129. In Bojrab MJ (ed): Pathophysiology in Small Animal Surgery. Lea & Febiger, Philadelphia, 1981

52. Schaer MJ: The use of regular insulin in the treatment of hyperkalemia in cats with urethral obstruction. J Am Anim Hosp Assoc 11:106, 1975

53. Shall WD, Greiner TP: Diseases of the gallbladder. p. 1456. In Ettinger SJ (ed): Textbook of Veterinary Internal Medicine II. WB Saunders, Philadelphia, 1983

54. Shields R: Digestion and absorption of food and fluids. In Wells CA (ed): Scientific Foundation of Surgery II. WB Saunders, Philadelphia, 1974

55. Stevenson S, Chew DJ, Kociba GJ: Torsion of the splenic pedicle in the dog: a review. J Am Anim Hosp Assoc 17(2):240, 1981

56. Tangner CH, Turrill JM, Hobson HP: Complications associated with proximal duodenal resection and cholecystoduodenostomy in two cats. Vet Surg 11(2):60, 1982

57. Toombs JP, Caywood DP, Lipowitz AJ, Stevens JB: Colonic perforation following neurosurgical procedures and corticosteroid therapy in four dogs. J Am Vet Med Assoc 177(1):68, 1980

58. Van Kruiningen HJ, Gregorie IC, Meuten DJ: Acute gastric dilation: a review of comparative aspects by species and a study in dogs and monkeys. J Am Anim Hosp Assoc 10:294, 1974

59. Wheaton LB, Strandberg JD, Hamilton SR, Bulkley GB: A comparison of three techniques for intraoperative prediction of small intestinal injury. J Am Anim Hosp Assoc 19(6):897, 1983

60. Wilson GP, Burt JK: Intussusception in the dog and cat: a review of 45 cases. J Am Anim Hosp Assoc 164:515, 1974

61. Wingfield WE: Acute gastric dilatation-volvulus syndrome. p. 149. In Bojrab MJ (ed): Current Techniques in Small Animal Surgery II. WB Saunders, Philadelphia, 1983
62. Wingfield WE, Betts CW, Rawlings CA: Pathophysiology associated with gastric dilatation-volvulus in the dog. J Am Anim Hosp Assoc 12:136, 1976
63. Wingfield WE, Betts CW, Greene RS: Operative techniques and recurrence rates associated with gastric volvulus in the dog. J Am Anim Hosp Assoc 16:427, 1975
64. Wolfe DA: Recurrent intestinal intussusceptions in the dog. J Am Vet Med Assoc 171(6):553, 1977
65. Wong PL: Pneumoperitoneum associated with splenic necrosis and clostridial peritonitis in a dog. J Am Anim Hosp Assoc 17(3):463, 1981
66. Wrigley RH, Reuter RE: Percutaneous cholecystography in normal dogs. Vet Radiol 23(6):239, 1982

9 | Emergency Treatment of Musculoskeletal Trauma

Erick L. Egger

While the dangling fractured leg or open joint is often the owner's primary concern, it is rarely life-threatening. The veterinarian must train himself to first overlook such obvious problems and accurately assess the patient's overall condition. Damage to the respiratory tract, such as pulmonary contusion, pneumothorax, and diaphragmatic hernia, is commonly seen with major trauma to the forelimb. Similarly, abdominal injuries such as splenic rupture or urinary tract laceration commonly occur with rear limb or pelvic trauma. Generalized shock can occur without gross outward signs. Failure to diagnose and accurately treat such conditions can complicate management or even prove fatal, particularly if tranquilization or anesthesia is used while applying splints or reducing luxations. Injuries to central and peripheral nervous tissues are easy to overlook, particularly if the animal has sustained multiple limb injuries. Likewise, a minimally displaced fracture or luxation of a proximal joint may not be apparent if the animal is not fully examined. Such oversights may affect not only the treatment regimen but the overall prognosis and the owner's willingness to proceed. The previous chapters of this book discuss the diagnosis and treatment of soft tissue injuries and systemic support of the traumatized patient. Such considerations should always be kept in mind.

On the other hand, the accurate and timely diagnosis and treatment of certain musculoskeletal and neurologic injuries is necessary for the overall success and economy of patient management. This chapter will discuss the diagnosis and treatment of such musculoskeletal and neurologic injuries.

FIRST AID FOR OWNERS

The owner or neighbor of the traumatized pet will often call requesting proper first aid information. The veterinarian or office personnel should caution such clients to protect themselves first since injured animals will often bite if in excessive pain or apprehensive. A calm, slow, reassuring approach should be advised, and the possibility of muzzling the patient, if necessary, is suggested. Next, significant bleeding must be controlled and open wounds protected from further contamination. A *clean* bandage, dressing, or even a large cloth applied with direct pressure will achieve both goals. The new disposable diapers work well and are commonly available. If the animal is nonambulatory, it should be gently slid onto a hard, flat surface such as a board or table leaf to allow transportation to veterinary facilities without causing additional displacement of neurologic or orthopedic injuries.

INITIAL PRESENTATION

When the injured animal is presented to the veterinary practice, the patient's overall condition must be thoroughly assessed and adequately managed. Open wounds should be covered or the previous dressing exchanged for a sterile dressing, and bleeding should be controlled with pressure or, in severe cases, hemostatic forceps. The musculoskeletal examination should begin away from the obvious fracture or injury. The animal that will not stand on three legs should be thoroughly scrutinized, particularly for central nervous system or contralateral orthopedic disease. Examination of the injured extremity should be the final step in the overall assessment. The skin should be carefully studied for wounds or devitalization that reduce or effectively eliminate the body's ability to impede bacterial invasion. The temperature of the limb distal to the injury should be assessed. A cold limb may indicate severe arterial compromise and extensive necrosis, particularly with open fractures and gunshot wounds. Edema distal to the injury is commonly seen and indicates the reduction of venous and lymphatic return. Usually such changes will resolve once lymphatic drainage and circulation have returned, but they do indicate effective disruption of circulation and tissue damage. Apparent nerve function is often abnormal in the injured extremity. Conscious proprioception and myotatic reflexes often reflect the mechanical inability of the musculoskeletal system to react in the normal manner. However, pain perception and motor function should be evaluated and any abnormalities investigated fully. Decreased pain perception or motor function in multiple limbs may indicate central nervous system injury and dictate spinal radiographic evaluation for spinal fractures or luxations. Such injuries will be discussed at length later in this chapter.

SPECIFIC INJURIES

Contusions

A contusion or bruise indicates capillary rupture and diffuse extravascular hemorrhage.[14] The free blood in tissues stimulates an inflammatory reaction with resultant edema. A contusion results from a direct blow to the body, such as occurs when an automobile bumper strikes the thigh or soft tissue is trapped between two hard objects such as the tibia and the pavement. Contusions usually present with a dark blue or black discoloration or abrasion of the skin. The haircoat may be absent or damaged. The injured area is often swollen and sensitive to palpation. Diagnosis is based on the clinical signs of skin discoloration, pain, and swelling. However, deep contusion of muscles may not result in skin changes. Characteristically, the pain and swelling of isolated contusions will resolve within a week. Contusions are often found concurrent with other traumatic injuries and must not be allowed to mask a more serious strain or sprain.

After the more serious injuries have been ruled out, contusions can be treated acutely with cold packs and direct pressure or compresive bandages, in order to limit further hemorrhage and edema formation. After 24 to 72 hours, moist heat and physiotherapy may be used to encourage vascularization that will help to clean up the inflammatory components and draw off edema. Confinement or tranquilization should be employed for several days to prevent reinjury of the contused area. Mild analgesics such as aspirin or butazolidin may be useful in more severe cases, but should not be allowed to obscure more severe injuries. The pain should be resolved within one week.

Strains

A strain is defined as damage to some part of the musculotendinous unit.[14] It can result from external trauma such as a severe blow or laceration or may reflect self-induced stretching or tearing from excessive or nonconditioned muscle contraction. The injury may occur in the muscle itself, or in the musculotendinous junction, the tendon, or the tendon's attachment to the bone at either end. Strains have been classified into first (mild), second (moderate), and third (severe) degree, based on the severity of the damage. The clinical signs of lameness and pain are often not apparent until the second or third day after injury and probably reflect the developing inflammatory process that will "clean up" the damaged tissue. First degree strains will be characterized by lameness and some pain on palpation. Second degree strains, likewise, cause pain or lameness and perhaps some swelling and muscular weakness. Third degree strains produce pain, lameness, swelling, and usually weakness. Severe third degree strains are essentially ruptures, and the animal will be unable to support weight or move the limb normally. Occasionally, lack of tissue can be palpated at the rupture site.

First and second degree strains can usually be managed conservatively. Rest of the injured musculotendinous unit, by confining or tranquilizing the

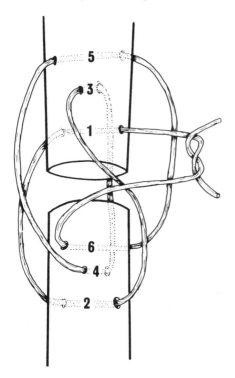

Fig. 9-1.   The pulley suture pattern for tendon and ligament repair consists of 3 continuous loops with the suture passed near (1)-far (2) middle (3)-middle (4) and far (5)-near (6) in relationship to the anastomotic site and each of the loops rotated 120° along the long axis.

animal, if necessary, is mandatory and should be maintained for 1 to 2 weeks, depending on the severity of the strain. Severe third degree strains and open lacerations often require surgical reconstruction to obtain a functional musculotendinous unit. This is most important in weightbearing units such as the Achilles complex or the triceps tendon. Closed ruptures are not emergencies but should be treated fairly acutely, since the damaged muscle will contract and fibrose, making surgical anastomosis difficult at a later time. Open lacerations should be debrided and the ends of the musculotendinous unit reanastomosed as soon as the animal can be safely anesthetized, in order to avoid further tissue devitalization and contraction. The Bunnell[17] or locking loop[1] suture patterns have been traditional for such purposes. However, recent experimental work has shown another suture pattern, the three-loop pulley pattern, to provide greater tensile strength and resist distraction of the sutured tendon ends.[3] A strong, nonabsorbable monofilament suture material such as nylon or polypropylene in the largest size that will atraumatically pass through the tissue should be used. The pattern consists of three loops placed in a near-far, middle–middle, and far–near orientation in relationship to the anastomosis site and rotated 120° along the tendon's long axis with each loop (Fig. 9-1). The paratenon is opposed with simple interrupted sutures of a small-sized, similar material. When repairing an injury of a multiple-component complex such as the Achilles, the individual components should be anastomosed separately, if possible. Such limbs should be supported with rigid external coaptation or external skeletal fixation in slight flexion or extension as needed to avoid tension on the sutured musculotendinous unit. The coaptation should be maintained for 3 to 4 weeks, followed by an additional 3 to 4 weeks of gradually increasing leg use. If a grossly contaminated or avulsion type of injury has occurred, the wound should be sterilely packed open, and closed after granulation has occurred or allowed to heal by second intention.

Sprains

A sprain is damage to a ligament.[14] Most sprains are caused by traumatic or athletic injuries, although some are associated with degenerative processes such as immune-mediated arthritis. Sprains are classified according to the severity of ligamentous damage and subsequent loss of supportive function. First degree sprains are associated with minimal ligamentous tearing but are often accompanied by intraligamentous hemorrhage that results in acute pain, lameness, and swelling. They do not result in palpable joint instability. Second degree sprains are associated with significant ligamentous tearing or stretching in addition to the bruising and hemorrhage. Since ligamentous elongation of 10 percent or less can result in loss of supporting function and can lead to secondary arthritic changes, such injuries should be promptly and aggressively treated. The acute clinical signs are similar to those of first degree sprain but will not rapidly resolve. Palpable instability may not be apparent, but stress radiography will often demonstrate widening of the affected joint. Third degree sprains represent severe tearing or total rupture of the ligament, resulting in loss of its supportive function. In addition to the clinical signs typical of less severe sprains, palpable instability is usually apparent. Radiographs should be used to confirm the injury and to rule out fractures or luxations.

First degree sprains can be treated conservatively, much like contusions and mild strains, with rest, acute cold packs to reduce hemorrhage and inflammation, and pain relievers. More severe sprains require aggressive management to provide functional support. If the injured ligament is not ensheathed with synovial membrane such as collateral ligaments, the ligament can heal primarily. This can be achieved in partially torn ligaments by external coaptation constructed to take the load off during weightbearing. Since ligaments heal slowly, support must be maintained for 3 to 4 weeks. Protection from any excessive load for another 4 to 8 weeks while healing matures and remodels is indicated. It is usually best to surgically treat severely torn or avulsed ligaments (third degree) to achieve the fastest and most satisfactory return to supportive function. The three-loop pulley pattern as described for tendon repair can be effectively used. Suturing of a severely traumatized ligament may not provide adequate support. For these cases, a large figure-of-eight suture of nylon or polypropylene can be placed between bone screws located at the ligament's attachments, in order to provide additional support while the tissues heal. Care must be taken not to overly tighten a ligament, since range of motion may be limited. Ligaments that have been torn away from the bone can be reattached using mattress sutures placed through the ligament and drawn

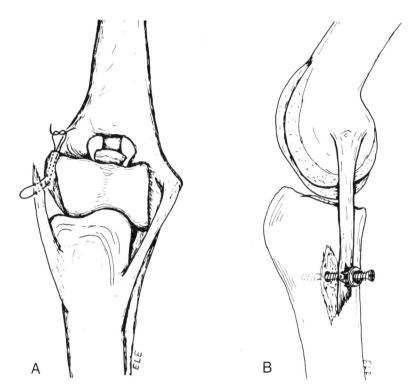

Fig. 9-2. Avulsed ligaments can be reattached with a mattress suture placed through the ligament and drawn through holes in the bone (A) or with a bone screw and spiked washer (B).

through holes drilled in the bone, or with a bone screw and spiked washer (Figs. 9-2A and 9-2B). Such repair should be supported either with external coaptation or external skeletal fixation for 4 to 6 weeks while the healing ligament gains strength.

Neurologic Injuries

Neurologic injuries can be divided into two groups depending upon the physiologic level at which they occur. Peripheral injuries occur in the nerve outside the central nervous system. Since such injuries interrupt the reflex arc, they are characterized by loss of muscle tone, hyporeflexia, and a varying extent of damage. *Neuroprazxia* is a stretching or bruising of the nerve fiber that results in some degree of dysfunction.[25] However, the fiber is viable, and normal function usually returns within a few days with little treatment. A good example of neuropraxia is bruising of the sciatic nerve with pelvic fractures. *Axonotmesis* is a more serious injury in which the nerve fiber is physically interrupted but the surrounding endoneurial tissue remains intact.[25] There is usually severe nerve dysfunction for an extended period of time, dependent upon the degree of damage. However, the nerve may be able to regenerate and function again. An example is a mild brachial plexus injury resulting from severe shoulder hyperextension and abduction. *Neuromesis* describes a complete disruption of the nerve fiber and supporting epineurium.[25] The loss of nerve function is complete and will not spontaneously return with conservative treatment. Severance of the radial nerve with an open supracondylar humeral fracture would be an example. Such nerves can return to function in some cases after surgical reanastomosis. The nerve will die back proximally to the closest ganglion and then slowly regenerate (approximately 1 cm per week) distally down the axon tube. The success of such procedures depends on the ability to achieve a good anastomosis and to avoid muscle contraction problems with physical therapy.

In the acute case with a clean severance, the anastomosis can be attempted using an epineural suture pattern.[25] The nerve ends should be closely examined and matched to achieve rotational alignment. Eight-0 monofilament nylon simple interrupted sutures are placed through the epineural sleeve, placing the first two sutures on opposite sides of the nerve. Additional sutures are then placed circumferentially at the widest intervals possible, consistent with achieving apposition of the nerve ends (Figs. 9-3A and 9-3B). Usually four to six sutures suffice. During the suturing process, the nerves should be handled only by the epineurium.

In severely contaminated, infected, or chronic injuries, the reanastomosis is probably best delayed until the surrounding tissues become healthy.[25] However, it is useful to tag the nerve ends with a bright, nonabsorbable suture material to facilitate identification and dissection at a later time. Resection and anastomosis of the nerve ends can be done after 3 to 5 weeks. However, such work requires magnification and microsurgical instrumentation and is beyond the scope of this paper. While such peripheral nerve repairs are possible, at least in some cases, they are expensive and time consuming, and require much dedication from both the veterinarian and the owner.

Central Nervous System Injuries

Central nervous system injuries involve either the brain or the spinal cord. This discussion will consider spinal cord injuries associated with vertebral column fractures or luxations, since they are often concurrent or confused with musculoskeletal damage. The clinical signs of central nervous system injuries vary with both the location and the severity of the injury. A cord lesion that occurs cranial to a reflex arc, leaving it intact, will result in upper motor neuron signs of muscles in that arc, such as hypertonia and hyperreflexia. This occurs because the modifying signals that descend from the brain are no longer able to reach the reflex arc. For example, a fracture of T-13 would result in exaggerated patellar myotatic reflexes, increased withdrawal reflexes of the hind limbs to toe pinch, and a generalized increased tone of the hind limb musculature. A central nervous system injury that occurs at the level of the reflex arc will result in lower motor neuron signs of hyporeflexia and hypotonia, as

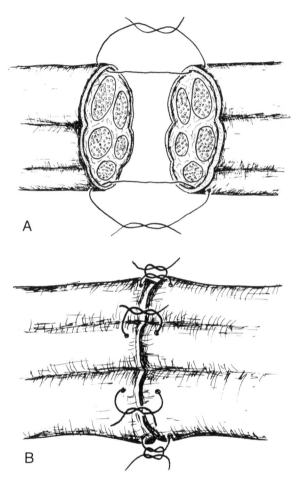

Fig. 9-3. Epineural anastomosis of a severed peripheral nerve begins with two sutures placed through the epineural sleeve to obtain axial alignment (A). Additional sutures are circumferentially placed to achieve apposition of the nerve ends (B).

described for the peripheral nerve injuries. An example would be a fracture–dislocation of L-4–5 resulting in a decrease in or the absence of patellar and withdrawal reflexes and flaccid hind limb musculature. An appropriately placed injury can result in both upper and lower motor neuron signs. For example, a luxation of C-6–C-7 would typically be characterized by hyporeflexia and hypotonia of the front limb and hyperreflexia and hypertonia of the hind limb. The severity of the lesion also affects the clinical signs. Generally, loss of conscious proprioception (posture or positioning), muscle paresis (weakness), muscle paralysis (loss of voluntary motion), and loss of deep pain perception (inability of the brain to perceive a noxious stimulus applied below the level of the injury) are felt to indicate increasingly severe injury.

The clinician must be sure in his examination that apparent deep pain perception reflects the response of the brain to stimuli, since withdrawal reflexes can be intact and result in limb motion caudal to a transected cord. If conscious perception of deep pain is present, at least some of the spinal cord is intact and the prognosis for recovery to at least partial function is fair, provided the injury is adequately stabilized to prevent progressive deterioration. If deep pain perception is not present, the spinal cord is severely injured or even transected. Since the cord has no ability to regenerate, the prognosis for such injuries is guarded at best and, depending on the owner's wishes, may either dictate euthanasia or an exploratory laminectomy in order to determine the extent of damage and to prognosticate recovery. Another clinical sign that occasionally appears is that of Schiff–Sherrington extensor rigidity.[8] This usually occurs with severe cord trauma in the midthoracic to lumbar area. It is characterized by foreleg extensor rigidity that appparently results from loss of the feedback that normally comes from the thoracolumbar portion of the cord and by flaccid paralysis of the hind limb, perhaps reflecting a "spinal shock" that interrupts the lower motor reflex arc. This clinical entity has traditionally carried a very poor prognosis. However, the clinician should be aware that this syndrome usually passes within several hours. Furthermore, local pain and excitement from bone and muscle injury will cause many less severely injured animals to hold the forelegs in extension, mimicking Schiff–Sherrington signs.

The appropriate method of treatment of central nervous system injury is highly controversial and varied. Medical treatment with large doses of steroids (dexamethasone 2 to 5 mg/kg) is aimed at reducing inflammation and stabilizing membranes. Diuretics (either mannitol 2 g/kg or furosemide 2 mg/kg) are used to physically reduce the swelling of the injured cord. Recently, the use of the opiate antagonist naloxone[11] and thyroid releasing hormone[12] have been explored as a means of preventing vascular spasm and decreasing cord hypoxia.[13] All of these medical treatments work best at the time of injury, necessitating expedient treatment to gain maximal benefit.

The debate about surgical stabilization of central nervous system injuries is also far from resolved. Most clinicians feel that conservative management with cage rest or external coaptation is appropriate for the less severe cases that remain stable.[25] Many surgeons now feel that the cases with more severe signs (muscle paralysis or questionable deep pain perception) or palpably or radiographically unstable fractures should be surgically stabilized. Many techniques have been developed, such as: dorsal spinal plating,[20] cross pinning,[15] and vertebral body plating.[27] The technique currently in use at Colorado State University involves dorsolateral placement of Steinmann pins in the vertebral bodies cranial and caudal to the fracture site. These pins are then stabilized with a "donut" of polymethyl methacrylate (Fig. 9-4). This technique provides excellent stabilization of even quite large dogs and can be applied anywhere along the spinal cord.[4,26] The use of a laminectomy has also been debated. Recent experience has shown that laminectomy may not significantly improve the prognosis of the case and may actually reduce the stability of the surgical repair.[4] However, laminectomy will allow more complete alignment of the fracture and visual assessment of the cord in cases with guarded prognosis. These surgical techniques are challenging at best and will not be specifically addressed here, other than by reference and to stress that they are most effective early in the course of injury. Consequently, such surgery or referral for surgery should be undertaken quickly for maximal benefit.

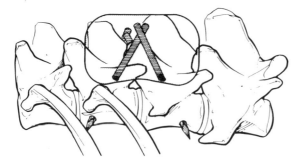

Fig. 9-4. Stabilization of the T-L junction with Steinmann pins and methyl methacrylate. (From Blass CE, Seim HB: Spinal fixation in dogs using Steinmann pins and methyl methacrylate. Vet Surg 13:203, 1984.)

FRACTURES

It has been said that no dog dies of a broken bone. For the most part that is true, and the clinician must be careful to accurately assess and treat more significant life-threatening problems. However, the appropriate and timely management of fractures can often enhance, speed, or even determine the success of bone healing and return to function. Fractures are currently described as being open or closed.[5] This terminology is more descriptive than the older nomenclature of compound versus simple. A closed fracture is one in which the skin remains intact, protecting the bone from the environment. The goals in emergency treatment of a closed fracture are to prevent the fracture from becoming open, to avoid damage to adjacent soft tissues (particularly nerves) and to reduce or prevent further hemorrhage and edema formation, making definitive fixation at a later time easier. These goals are best achieved in distal limb fractures (below the stifle or elbow) with a temporary compressive dressing (Robert Jones bandage).

Proximal limb fractures are more difficult to stabilize with external coaptation, have greater muscle mass to act as padding, and can often be best managed acutely with cage rest. If the animal must be bandaged for transport or management of other problems, the compressive wrap previously described can be extended proximally over the shoulder or hip, incorporating the trunk, to become a spica. Care must be used not to embarrass respiration with forelimb spicas or to compromise urination in the male dog with hind limb spicas. These bandages can be maintained for 3 to 5 days while the animal is stabilized or transferred for definitive fracture fixation. In general, tranquilization should be avoided, since it tends to cause hypotension and makes assessment of neurologic conditions more difficult or impossible.

Open Fracture

An open fracture is defined as one in which the fractured bone has been exposed to the external environment.[5,23] In type I open fractures, the wound in the skin is made by the end of the fragment protruding; consequently, there is relatively little soft tissue injury and contamination of the deep wound. In type II open fractures, the skin wound is made by an outside agent which also contaminates the fracture site. The degree of soft tissue injury and contamination can vary from mild, as from a bite wound, to serious, as that incurred by a gunshot in which the mass of the bullet causes radiating soft tissue damage and carries foreign material that remains in the wound. A type III open fracture is associated with extensive soft tissue damage or loss and wound contamination. The fracture is often comminuted and may have defects resulting from fragment loss. The bone may be highly contaminated and stripped of its soft tissue attachments and blood supply. This type of fracture often results from skidding or dragging on a roadway, resulting in avulsion or shearing of soft tissue and bone.

The duration of the injury must also be considered in the management and prognosis of open fractures.[23] During the first 6 to 8 hours, the wound is considered contaminated. Bacteria are present but have not had the opportunity to multiply and spread through the adjacent tissues. If the wound is appropriately treated during this "golden period," clinical infection should not occur. However, once the bacteria have become established, the wound must be considered infected. Infection can extend the soft tissue and osseous damage, potentially converting a relatively simple type I fracture into a difficult type III or perhaps resulting in fixation failure and nonunion. All open fractures must be considered contaminated.

The overall goals of open fracture treatment are to treat the wound to avoid additional contamination, to avert conversion of contamination to infection, or, if the wound is already infected, to stabilize the fracture and manage the infection so that bone healing can proceed.

Initial Treatment of Open Fractures

The initial treatment of open fractures can be begun by the owner. Since the majority of fracture infections result from bacteria found to be indigenous to veterinary clinics and not present in the outside environment,[23] simply covering the wound with a clean cloth will reduce the amount of contamination that will have to be dealt with later. Once the patient has been presented to a clinical facility, the cloth should be replaced with a sterile gauze dressing. When initial assessment and shock therapy have been accomplished, the hair on the fractured limb can be clipped and removed. Coating the hair on the periphery of the wound with sterile water-soluble lubricating gel will allow removal of the hair while avoiding further contamination. Radiographs of the fractured limb should be performed and examined to help to formulate the prognosis and a plan for fixation.

As soon as is safely possible, the open fracture should be debrided and stabilized. This will usually require general anesthesia or, in hind limb cases, tranquilization and an epidural block. Any final clipping can then be performed before uncovering the wound. The patient should be moved to a clean area or, preferably, to the operating room, and the intact skin can be prepared as for normal aseptic surgery. Cap, mask, and gloves should be donned prior to removing the dressing and performing the initial wound cleansing. A nonirritating solution such as chlorhexidine in saline should be used. The wound should be cultured to determine the contaminating organism and to direct postoperative antibiotic therapy.

Debridement

After the veterinarian has donned a sterile gown and changed gloves, the wound is thoroughly debrided. Debridement means removal of all foreign material and contaminated or dead tissue. In many open fractures, it may be necessary to enlarge the wound for exposure. This must be balanced against the deleterious effect of soft tissue damage and vascular compromise inherent in such exposure. Copious irrigation and suction (lavage) of the wound with an isotonic solution such as normal saline or Ringer's solution will help to remove the degenerative material. Antiseptics or antibiotics used to be added to the irrigation solution, but the current preference is to use large volumes of lavage solution, that physically dilutes the contaminating organisms to a number insufficient to establish an infection. A pulsating irrigation delivery system can be effectively used to help lavage. A significant amount of pressure is used in order to mechanically remove devitalized tissue, microorganisms, and foreign material. There is some concern that high-pressure irrigation drives contamination deeper into surrounding normal tissues.[23] However, it is felt that this potential disadvantage is outweighed by the advantages of a high-pressure technique.

Fracture Stabilization

It is important to emphasize that an infected fracture will heal if it is adequately stabilized. The infection can then be controlled. An unstable, infected fracture will not heal and will remain infected, because fracture motion disturbs the vascular ingrowth that is ultimately responsible for both fracture healing and infection control. Consequently, external coaptation is rarely an adequate primary fixation for open fractures, since it fails to provide the rigidity needed for rapid revascularization, particularly if wound drainage requires bandage changes.[23]

Intramedullary pin fixation of open fractures is usually avoided, since it introduces a metallic foreign body through the contaminated or infected fracture into the length of the medullary cavity. The pin will often serve as a haven for bacterial proliferation and can spread infection throughout the bone. As the osteomyelitis causes bone lysis, pin purchase fails and an infected nonunion commonly results. Even if the fracture heals, the pin usually serves as a nidus for continuing osteomyelitis until it is removed, and such removal can be very diffciult if the pin is buried.

Bone screw and plate fixation provides very stable and extended fixation, if sufficient bone exists for adequate screw purchase. Consequently, such fixation is useful for the extremely comminuted fracture for which protracted

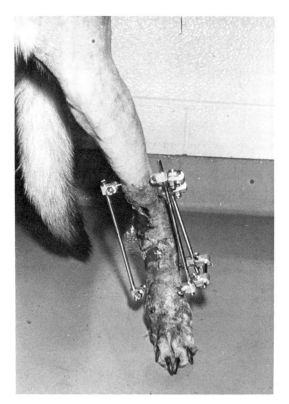

Fig. 9-5. External skeletal fixation can be used to stabilize open fractures without placing implants in the damaged tissue, yet still allows easy access for wound management.

healing is predicted. Extensive surgical exposure is required for placement, usually resulting in some additional vascular damage and the presence of a large metallic implant in contact with the contaminated wound, which often results in continued infection until the implants can be removed. Unfortunately, the equipment and additional training necessary to use plates and the non-reusable, expensive nature of the implants themselves preclude their use in many practices.

External skeletal fixation is particularly well-suited for fixation of open fractures, since the fixation pins can often be placed through intact soft tissue into undamaged bone, thus avoiding the spread of contamination from the wound and minimizing surgically induced vascular damage (Fig. 9-5). Newly described design configurations[10] and refined techniques of application have recently increased the rigidity and durability of external skeletal fixation[2], allowing it to be used on many unstable fractures where fragments are too short or comminuted for plate and screw fixation. In addition, external skeletal fixation is relatively easy to apply and requires little specialized equipment. Furthermore, the connecting clamps and bars of the apparatus can be reused often, resulting in an economical and practical form of fixation for the general practitioner.

Bone Graft

Most open fractures take longer to heal than similar closed fractures, due to the vascular damage inherent in such injuries. Cancellous bone placed in such fractures induces callus formation and speeds fracture healing. A cancellous bone graft will be incorporated in most vascular wounds.[23] Such a graft rarely becomes infected; however, if it does, cancellous bone will liquefy and drain out, causing no damage. Cancellous graft can be collected for front leg fractures from the craniolateral aspect of the humeral greater tubercle. For hindlimb application, the graft can be obtained from the medial proximal tibia and the craniodorsal ilial wing. To obtain the maximal biologic effect, the graft should be collected and placed in the fracture site after debridement, lavage, and stabilization. However, to avoid inducing infection at the donor site, it may be advisable to collect the graft and store it in a glass bowl covered with saline or blood moistened gauze sponges before a contaminated fracture is approached. Alternately, the surgeon can change gloves and use additional equipment to collect a graft aseptically when needed.

Graft collection is usually done through a short (1–2 cm) skin and fascial incision directly over the bone of the humerus or tibia. A somewhat longer skin incision (5–8 cm) and muscle separation is required to approach the dorsal ilium. A self-retaining retractor (Gelpi or Weitlander) is useful to maintain this limited exposure. A Steinmann pin (1/4 inch for most dogs, 5/32 inch for cats and very small dogs) and hand chuck is then used to create a hole through the outer cortical bone into the metaphysis. The pin is preferable to a trephine or drill bit because its sharp point prevents slippage on the cortical surface, and the twisting wrist motion does not engage adjacent soft tissues. A bone curette nearly as large as the pin is then used to collect the graft. Again, a twisting wrist motion is used to cut the cancellous bone from its bed. The cancellous bone obtained is packed in any cracks or defects that persist and along the fracture line after the fracture is reduced. When the wound is not to be closed, the cancellous graft should be covered with sterile saline soaked gauze packs until the granulation tissue covers the wound. In very avascular or purulent wounds, the fracture should be debrided and stabilized, and cancellous graft application delayed for 10 to 14 days while granulation tissue proliferates enough to provide vascular support for the graft.[16]

Cortical bone grafts are generally contraindicated in acute, significantly contaminated or infected fractures because of a high incidence of graft infection and sequestration. The use of a massive cancellous graft to fill defects, accepting mild shortening of the bone, and obtaining stable reduction generally gives the best results. Delayed cortical grafting can be attempted, but infection is still a common sequela.

Closure

If the contamination and vascular damage are mild as in a type I open fracture and the site can be completely debrided, a primary closure of the wound may be attempted. Incorporation of a Penrose drain in the wound prevents fluid accumulation and allows monitoring of the fracture site but requires care to avoid retrograde infection. Interrupted suture patterns are useful because they can be partially removed to encourage additional drainage, if needed.

My experience with inflow/outflow irrigation systems in small animals has been unsatisfactory. The mechanics of keeping tubes functional with uncooperative patients is difficult, and infection around the tubing is common. Generally, if there is a question about the completeness of debridement, the wound is packed open. A pad of sterile saline soaked gauze sponges placed in the wound and covered with a bulky absorbent cotton bandage works well. The bandage should be changed in a clean environment using aseptic technique every 3 to 4 days until granulation tissue covers the bone. Lavage of the wound with sterile saline will help to remove accumulated debris. During these bandage changes, the wound may have to be debrided of both necrotic soft tissue and cortical bone which will not incorporate into the developing granulation tissue. Once granulation is complete, the wound can be left uncovered to heal by second intention or can be closed with a skin graft.

Broad-spectrum antibiotics should be used during the initial treatment of open fractures; then more specific drug selection should be directed by fracture healing or drainage culture results. Topical antibiotics are generally not indicated, since any vascularized tissue will receive systemic protection, and avascular tissues should be debrided or allowed to liquefy and drain away.

JOINTS

Joint Infections

Joint infection (septic arthritis) is an extremely serious problem because the infectious agents and the degenerative products directly attack and destroy articular cartilage.[28]

A septic arthritis of hematogenous origin implies that the infectious agent arrived at the joint through its blood supply. This type of infection is uncommonly seen in small animals. It is usually associated with septicemia and commonly involves multiple joints. In the very young dog, septic arthritis can originate from an umbilical infection or a generalized pyoderma. In the older animal it can originate from endocarditis, periodontal disease, or prostatic abscessation.

Joint infections of nonhematogenous origin are generally caused by penetrating wounds and may be associated with a foreign body.

The clinical appearance of joint infection resembles any other active infection, with pain, heat, swelling, and fever apparent. Consequently, microscopic examination of joint fluid may be necessary to differentiate an abscess near a joint from a joint infection. However, the tap should be performed through healthy tissue to avoid contamination of a healthy joint.

The treatment of the problem centers around two modalities: appropriate antibiotic therapy and removal of the injurious material from the joint space.

Antibiotic therapy should begin as soon as possible. A broad-spectrum drug or a combination such as intravenous ampicillin and intramuscular gentamicin that will quickly reach effective systemic therapeutic levels is desired. Cultures of the joint fluid should be performed but often demonstrate no bacterial growth. A culture of synovial membrane commonly gives positive results and can be used to definitively direct antibiotic selection.

The method of removing exudate from the joint depends on the chronicity of the infection. If treated acutely (within 24 to 48 hours), the joint can be thoroughly lavaged with large volumes of isotonic solution, using injection needles. The hair around the joint should be clipped and the skin surgically prepared to prevent further contamination. Usually one needle is attached to an intravenous administration set or a large syringe to provide inflow, and one or two needles are placed across the joint to provide outflow. The lavage should be continued until the exiting fluid is clear and acellular. Periodic manipulation of the joint through its range of motion will help to distribute the solution throughout the joint space. Addition of antibiotics to the solution is usually not indicated, since absorption is unpredictable and many antibiotics will damage articular cartilage. The lavage cycle should be repeated two to three times a day until the joint fluid remains clear and acellular between cycles.

Within a few days the infected fluid will form a fibrin clot that cannot be removed by closed lavage.[7] Likewise, joints containing foreign bodies will remain chronically infected. These joints need to be surgically explored and debrided of organized clots or foreign bodies. More chronic joint infections cause synovial proliferation. The infectious agent becomes sequestered from the antibiotic and lavage therapy and acts as a chronic nidus. Synovectomy has been reported as a means of managing such chronic infections in horses.[18] The appropriate manner of closing the surgical wound is much like that for open fractures. If the wound can be debrided and lavaged clean, it can be closed primarily or over a Penrose drain. If the chronicity or severity of the problem precludes converting it to an aseptic field, it should be packed open and allowed to drain and granulate until it can be safely closed after 10 to 14 days. The bandage should be changed every 3 to 4 days and the joint thoroughly lavaged at that time.

Joint Luxation

Traumatic luxation of a joint implies that the ligaments or tendons that stabilize that joint and the joint capsule that surrounds it have been traumatically stretched or torn so that the articular surfaces of the bones involved are no longer in contact. A congenital luxation implies that the articular surfaces of the joint have never been in proper alignment, and it is usually associated with osseous malformation or ligamentous hypoplasia. The direction of the luxation is described by the position of the distal articular component in relation to the proximal component.

Traumatic joint luxations should be reduced and stabilized as soon as possible, taking into consideration the patient's overall condition, for a number of reasons. Delay in reduction allows muscles that surround the joint to contract and even fibrose in chronic cases, making reduction difficult. Delay of reduction gives the hemarthrosis, which usually occurs within the joint, time to accumulate and organize into a fibrin clot that can physically prevent complete reduction. Finally, the articular cartilage itself will be damaged while luxated. It will not be bathed in the synovial fluid that provides its nutrition. It will also be rubbing against the opposite cartilage. Forelimb joint luxations must be performed under general anesthesia to overcome muscle contraction and avoid pain. Short acting barbiturate or gas anesthesia works well. Hip luxations can be reduced under general anesthesia; alternately, epidural anesthesis provides excellent muscle relaxation; it is particularly useful in larger animals.

Open luxations are luxations with an open wound from the environment to the joint space. In addition to early reduction and stabilization, these injuries require appropriate management, as previously described for joint infection and open fracture.

Specific Joint Luxations

Shoulder. The shoulder joint is stabilized partially by four cuff muscles: the supraspinatus cranially, the infraspinatus laterally, the teres minor caudally, and the subscapularis medially.[22] In addition, there are medial and lateral thickenings in the joint capsule that provide a variable degree of collateral ligament effect.[6] Medial traumatic luxations are most common in toy and small breed dogs, while lateral luxations are more common in larger dogs.[5] These traumatic luxations can often be managed by closed reduction within a few days of injury. In general, flexion of both the shoulder and the elbow joints relieves muscle pull. A combination of internal rotation with adduction for medial luxations or external rotation with abduction for lateral luxations will achieve reduction. Following radiographic confirmation of reduction, the medial luxation case should be placed in a Velpeau sling which forces the humeral head laterally, and an over the shoulder spica splint should be used to support a reduced lateral luxation. Traumatic luxations that cannot be reduced or reluxate, or congenitally unstable shoulders, such as are seen in toy poodles or shelties, can be surgically stabilized by reefing of the joint capsule[19] and transposition of the biceps tendon laterally for lateral luxation[5] or by medial transposition of part of the supraspinatus tendon for medial luxation.[6]

Traumatic Elbow Luxations. The interlocking anatomy of the elbow makes it relatively resistant to luxation. Consequently, the severity of trauma necessary to cause luxation predisposes to lateral condylar fracture instead, particularly if the limb were in extension when injured. Luxations usually occur when the elbow is flexed, thus freeing the anconeal process from the supracondylar fossa. The proximal ulna almost always displaces laterally due to the smaller lateral humeral condyle. Many such luxations can be managed with closed reduction if done within a few days of injury. The elbow is flexed to reduce muscle pull and traction applied to free the anconeal process. The forelimb is internally rotated to catch the anconeal process inside the lateral humeral epicondyle and the joint extended to lock it in place. Additional internal rotation and medial force on the radial head will force it back into reduction with the lateral humeral condyle. Once reduced, the collateral ligament should be checked by rotation of the paw with the paw and elbow held at 90° flexion.[5] Lateral rotation of the paw significantly beyond 45° implies medial collateral injury. Medial rotation significantly beyond 70° implies lateral collateral injury. If both collaterals appear intact, the limb should be immobilized with the elbow held in moderate extension by a soft padded bandage for 7 to 10 days. If one of the collaterals has been damaged but the joint remains stable, immobilization in extension with a lateral splint for two to three weeks may provide adequate support to allow healing. However, if the elbow is unstable after reduction, or, the patient is large or active, surgical repair of damaged ligaments as previously described is indicated. After surgical collateral repair, the limb should be supported in a lateral or spica splint for three to four weeks. Following any bandaging of the forelimb, passive range of motion exercises may be necessary to reestablish elbow movement.

Carpus.   True luxations of the antebrachial carpal joint are rarely seen and are usually associated with severe trauma, multiple ligamentous ruptures, and articular damage. Usually such cases can only be satisfactorily stabilized by pancarpal arthrodesis.[24] Subluxation of the carpus is occasionally seen and is associated with unilateral collateral ligament rupture. Such injuries can best be documented by stress radiography which will demonstrate at what level the deficiency has occurred. Treatment is undertaken as previously described, by primary suturing of the ligament and support with screws and figure of eight sutures. Shearing injuries of the carpus occur when a limb is in contact with an abrasive surface such as an asphalt or concrete roadway. Skin, ligamentous support, articular cartilage, and even bone are commonly ground away. If a significant portion of the joint articular surface is removed, primary arthrodesis offers the best prognosis. However, less damaged joints can often be saved by aggressive surgical treatment.[9] Following debridement and lavage as described for open fractures, small bone screws are placed in the approximate location of collateral ligament attachment. Figure-of-eight sutures of large, nonabsorbable material placed around the screw heads are then used to replace the missing ligaments. External skeletal fixation is often used to provide additional uninterrupted support. The wound is packed open with sterile gauze sponges and additionally debrided every 3 days as needed until the granulation covers the abraded surface and the implants. The external skeletal fixation should be removed in 3 to 4 weeks and the limb protected with soft padded bandaging for an additional 3 to 4 weeks.

Hyperextension of the carpus is actually a severe sprain or rupture of the palmar fibrocartilage that results in loss of palmar support and hyperextension of the middle carpal or carpometacarpal joints. In smaller, quiet breeds, such acute injuries can occasionally be managed by palmar support for 4 weeks.[16] However, if the injury has become chronic or is seen in larger, active dogs, the fibrosis that occurs with splintage will usually not suffice, and the hyperextension will recur.[16] Partial carpal arthrodesis of these lower joints, stabilized with external coaptation[16] or pin fixation,[5] will provide satisfactory support yet allow continued antebrachial carpal motion.

Hip Luxations. Luxation of the coxofemoral joint is associated with rupture of the round ligament and partial tearing of the joint capsule. The femoral head can be displaced in one of several directions. A craniodorsal luxation in which the femoral head lies cranial and dorsal to the acetabulum is the most common hip luxation, probably due to the weightbearing and propulsive forces in that direction. In addition, contraction of the gluteal muscles draws the femur in a cranial and dorsal direction. Caudodorsal luxations are rarely seen and are usually associated with a severe force that has avulsed the gluteal muscle attachments from the trochanter. Some risk of sciatic nerve damage is inherent both due to the severity of the trauma and the position of the head in the sciatic notch. Ventral luxation, in which the femoral head is displaced distally, usually into the obturator foramen, is an infrequent injury. This variation occurs when a limb is caught and pulled ventral to the body or severely abducted.

The clinical signs of hip luxation include lameness, pain on palpation, apparent decrease or increase of limb length, and internal or external rotation, depending upon the direction of femoral head luxation. Also, the distance from the greater trochanter to the tuber ischii will vary from the contralateral normal. However, these clinical signs cannot be distinguished from those of femoral head and neck fractures or certain acetabular fractures. Additionally, the possible presence of hip dysplasia or round ligament avulsion fractures that essentially preclude effective closed reduction mandate that all coxofemoral luxations be adequately radiographed.

Many coxofemoral luxations can be successfully managed with early closed reduction and external support, assuming that osseous anatomy is normal. The gluteal muscles go into spasm with time, making manipulation more difficult. The blood clot usually present in the acetabulum will organize into a fibrotic mass, making femoral head seating even more difficult. Consequently, reduction of such luxations should be done as soon as is safely possible.

Craniodorsal luxations are reduced by applying distal traction and external rotation to the lower limb and countertraction around the pelvis, while pulling the femoral head distal to the acetabular rim. Internal rotation of the leg and medial pressure upon the greater trochanter is then used to force the head deep into the acetabulum. With a medially-directed force on the greater trochanter, passive range of motion is then used to work the blood and the fibrin clot out of the joint. The limb is then placed in a modified Ehmer sling that holds the femur in abduction and internal rotation, maximizing femoral head seating, for 5 to 14 days, depending on stability of the hip after reduction and the size and activity of the patient.

Ventral luxations can often be reduced with adduction and external or internal rotation while pulling distally on the limb to disengage the femoral head from the obturator foramen. This allows the femoral head to snap dorsally into the acetabulum. Once reduced, the head should be seated as previously described with a medial force applied to the greater trochanter and range of motion exercises. The limb is secured to the opposite hind limb with tape hobbles to prevent abduction for 5 to 10 days.

Coxofemoral luxations that cannot be reduced by closed manipulation or that easily reluxate often have severe joint capsule tearing or the joint capsule is entrapped between the femoral head and acetabulum. They require open reduction and surgical stabilization beyond the scope of this discussion. However, they can be delayed for several days, if necessary, until the patient's general condition will allow longer anesthesia.

Stifle Luxation.   The stifle joint is essentially a hinge stabilized entirely by ligamentous support. Consequently, luxation of the stifle implies significant ligamentous disruption. Any hope for return to joint function requires surgical reconstruction of these ligaments. Alternatively, arthrodesis of the stifle can be used to achieve a pain-free, useful limb.[5]

Tarsus.   The tarsal joint is supported by collateral ligaments and suffers injuries similar to those of the carpus. Total luxations usually require arthrodesis, while collateral ligament disruptions associated with subluxation can be surgically stabilized as previously described. Similar to the carpus, shearing injuries of the tarsus can often be managed surgically by debridement, lavage, and suture stabilization around bone screws, with external coaptation or external skeletal fixation support.[21]

REFERENCES

1. Aron DN: A "new" tendon stitch. J Am Anim Hosp Assoc 17:587, 1981
2. Aron DN, Toombs JP: Updated principles of external skeletal fixation. Comp Cont Educ 6:845, 1984
3. Berg RJ, Egger EL: Comparison of the pulley and locking loop suture patterns for repair of canine tendons and ligaments. Submitted to Vet Surg
4. Blass CE, Seim HB: Spinal fixation in dogs using Steinmann pins and methyl methacrylate. Vet Surg 73:203, 1984
5. Brinker WO, Piermattei DL, Flo GL. pp. 2, 330, 354, 375, 396. In Handbook of Small Animal Orthopedics and Fracture Treatment. W B Saunders Co, Philadelphia, 1983
6. Craig E, Hohn RB, Anderson WD: Surgical stabilization of traumatic medial shoulder dislocation. J Am Anim Hosp Assoc 16:93, 1980
7. Daniel D et al: Lavage of septic joints in rabbits: effects of chondrolysis. J Bone Jt Surg 58A:393, 1976
8. DeLahunta A: p. 180. In Veterinary Neuroanatomy and Clinical Neurology. W B Saunders, Philadelphia, 1977
9. Earley T: Canine carpal ligament injuries. Vet Clin North Am 8:183, 1978
10. Egger EL: Static strength evaluation of six external skeletal fixation configurations. Vet Surg 12:130, 1983
11. Faden AI et al: Endorphins in experimental spinal injury: therapeutic effect of naloxone. Ann Neurol 10:326, 1981
12. Faden AI et al: Thyrotropin-releasing hormone improves neurologic recovery after spinal trauma in cats. N Engl J Med 305:1063, 1981

13. Faden AI, Jacobs TP, Holaday JW: Opiate antagonist improves neurologic recovery after spinal injury. Science 211:493, 1981
14. Farrow CS: Sprain, strain, and contusion. Vet Clin North Am 8:169, 1978
15. Gage ED: A new method of spinal fixation in the dog. VM/SAC 64:295, 1969
16. Gambardella PC, Griffiths RC: Treatment of hyperextension injuries of the canine carpus. Comp Cont Educ 4:127, 1982
17. Knecht CD et al: p. 45. In Fundamental Techniques in Veterinary Surgery. W B Saunders, Philadelphia, 1975
18. Leitch M: Diagnosis and treatment of septic arthritis in the horse. J Am Vet Med Assoc 175:701, 1979
19. Lippincott CL: Reefing of the shoulder joint. A technique to surgically restore the integrity of a luxated scapulohumeral articulation in the dog. VM/SAC 66:695, 1971
20. Lumb WV, Brasmer TH: Improved spinal plates and hypothermia as adjuncts to spinal surgery. J Am Vet Med Assoc 157:338, 1970
21. Matthiesan DT: Tarsal injuries in the dog and cat. Comp Cont Educ 5:548, 1983
22. Miller ME, Christensen GC, Evans HE: pp. 240–243. In Anatomy of the Dog. 2nd Ed. W B Saunders, Philadelphia, 1979
23. Nunamaker DM: Treatment of open fractures in small animals. Comp Cont Educ 1:66, 1979
24. Parker RB, Brown SG, Wind AP: Pancarpal arthrodesis in the dog: a review of forty-five cases. Vet Surg 10:35, 1981
25. Rodkey WG, Carbaud HE: Peripheral nerve injury and repair. pp. 24–29. In Bojrab MJ (ed): Current Techniques in Small Animal Surgery. 2nd Ed. Lea & Febiger, Philadelphia, 1983
26. Rouse GP, Milton JI: The use of methyl methacrylate for spinal stabilization. J Am Anim Hosp Assoc 11:418, 1975
27. Swaim SF: Vertebral body plating for spinal immobilization. J Am Vet Med Assoc 158:1683, 1971
28. Warning TL: Acute infectious arthritis and wounds of joints. pp. 963–986. In Crenshaw AH (ed): Campbell's Operative Orthopedics, 5th Ed. C V Mosby Co, St. Louis, 1971

Index

Page numbers followed by f represent figures; those followed by t represent tables.